Essentials of
Nuclear Medicine
Physics and
Instrumentation

Essentials of Nuclear Medicine Physics and Instrumentation

Rachel A. Powsner, MD

Associate Professor of Radiology
Boston University School of Medicine
Director, Division of Nuclear Medicine
Department of Radiology
Boston Veterans Administration Healthcare System
Boston, MA, USA

Matthew R. Palmer, PhD

Medical Physicist
Department of Radiology
Beth Israel Deaconess Medical Center
Assistant Professor of Radiology
Harvard Medical School
Boston, MA, USA

Edward R. Powsner, MD

Former Chief, Nuclear Medicine Service
Veterans Administration Hospital
Allen Park, MI
Former Professor and Associate Chairman
Department of Pathology
Michigan State University
East Lansing, MI, USA

THIRD EDITION

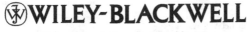

A John Wiley & Sons, Ltd., Publication

This edition first published 2013, © 2013 by John Wiley & Sons, Ltd

Wiley-Blackwell is an imprint of John Wiley & Sons, formed by the merger of Wiley's global Scientific, Technical and Medical business with Blackwell Publishing.

Registered office: John Wiley & Sons Ltd, The Atrium, Southern Gate, Chichester, West Sussex, PO19 8SQ, UK

Editorial offices: 9600 Garsington Road, Oxford, OX4 2DQ, UK
 The Atrium, Southern Gate, Chichester, West Sussex, PO19 8SQ, UK
 111 River Street, Hoboken, NJ 07030-5774, USA

For details of our global editorial offices, for customer services and for information about how to apply for permission to reuse the copyright material in this book please see our website at www.wiley.com/wiley-blackwell

Library of Congress Cataloging-in-Publication Data

Powsner, Rachel A.
 [Essentials of nuclear medicine physics]
 Essentials of nuclear medicine physics and instrumentation / Rachel A. Powsner, MD, associate professor of radiology, Boston University School of Medicine, director, Division of Nuclear Medicine, Department of Radiology, Boston Veterans Administration Healthcare System, Boston, MA, USA, Matthew R. Palmer, PhD, medical physicist, Department of Radiology, Beth Israel Deaconess Medical Center, assistant professor of radiology, Harvard Medical School, Boston, MA, USA, Edward R. Powsner, MD, former chief, Nuclear Medicine Service, Veterans Administration Hospital, Allen Park, MI, former professor and associate chairman, Department of Pathology, Michigan State University, East Lansing, MI, USA. – Third edition.
  pages cm
 Includes bibliographical references and index.
 ISBN 978-0-470-90550-0 (pbk. : alk. paper)
 1. Nuclear medicine. 2. Medical physics. I. Palmer, Matthew R., 1958– II. Powsner, Edward R., 1926– III. Title.
 R895.P69 2013
 616.07′575–dc23

                    2012047264

A catalogue record for this book is available from the British Library.

Wiley also publishes its books in a variety of electronic formats. Some content that appears in print may not be available in electronic books.

Cover Design: Michael Rutkowski
Cover Illustration: (top) © Jeja/iStockphoto; (bottom) courtesy of Rachel A. Powsner

Set in 9/12 pt Photina by Toppan Best-set Premedia Limited, Hong Kong

Contents

Preface, vii

Acknowledgments, viii

1. Basic Nuclear Medicine Physics, 1

2. Interaction of Radiation with Matter, 21

3. Formation of Radionuclides, 32

4. Nonscintillation Detectors, 41

5. Scintillation Detectors, 60

6. Imaging Instrumentation, 73

7. Single-photon Emission Computed
   Tomography, 91

8. Positron Emission Tomography, 103

9. X-ray Computed Tomography, 119

10. Hybrid Imaging Systems: PET-CT and
    SPECT-CT, 129

11. Image Reconstruction, Processing,
    and Display, 134

12. Information Technology, 161

13. Quality Control, 168

14. Radiation Biology, 185

15. Radiation Dosimetry, 197

16. Radiation Safety, 205

17. Management of Nuclear Event
    Casualties, 212
    with Kevin Donohoe, MD

Appendix A: Common Nuclides, 224

Appendix B: Major Dosimetry for Common
            Radiopharmaceuticals, 225

Appendix C: Sample Calculations of the
            S Value, 226

Appendix D: Guide to Nuclear Regulatory
            Commission Publications, 228

Appendix E: Recommended Reading by Topic, 231

Index, 232

Preface

After years of postgraduate training, many physicians have forgotten some (or most) of their undergraduate and high school physics and may find submersion into nuclear physics somewhat daunting. This book begins with a very basic introduction to nuclear physics and the interactions of radiation and matter. It then proceeds with discussions of nuclear medicine instrumentation used for production of nuclides, measurement of doses, surveying radioactivity, and imaging (including SPECT, PET, CT, PET-CT, and SPECT-CT). An introduction to information technology is followed by a chapter on instrumentation quality control. The final chapters cover radiation biology, radiation safety, and radiation accidents.

Numerous illustrations are included. They are highly schematic and are designed to illustrate concepts rather than represent scale models of their subjects. This text is intended for radiology residents, cardiology fellows, nuclear medicine fellows, nuclear medicine technology students, and others interested in an introduction to concepts in nuclear medicine physics and instrumentation.

Rachel A. Powsner
Matthew R. Palmer
Edward R. Powsner

Acknowledgments

The authors would like to thank the following individuals for their help with this edition: Anupma Jati, MD, kindly critiqued the CT dosimetry section of the text. On the topic of quality control, Gary Murphy, RT, was most helpful with CT-related questions and Kandace Craft, RTN, and Chris Lindsey, FSE, answered queries about PET-CT. P. Satish Nair, PhD, generously made comments on the dosimetry chapter and David Drum, MD, also reviewed this portion and answered numerous questions about radiation safety and dosimetry. We wish to thank J. Anthony Parker, MD, for his helpful comments on the topic of cancer induction from low-dose ionizing radiation as well as serving as a reference for an assortment of specific questions relating to the text. The authors also gratefully acknowledge Dr. Kevin Donohoe, who kindly shared his expertise and took the time to review and supplement the material on radiation accidents in the current and preceding edition of this text. Since this edition incorporates text from prior editions, the authors would like to thank the following individuals for their help with the second edition: Stephen Moore, PhD, on the topic of SPECT processing, including iterative reconstruction; Fred Fahey, DSc, on PET instrumentation; and Robert Zimmerman, MSEE, on gamma camera quality control and the physics of crystal scintillators. In addition, Dr. Frank Masse generously reviewed the material on radiation accidents and Mark Walsh, CHP, critiqued the radiation safety text.

We would also like to thank the following individuals for their help in reviewing portions of the first edition during its preparation: David Rockwell, MD, Maura Dineen-Burton, CNMT, Dipa Patel, MD, Alfonse Taghian, MD, Hernan Jara, PhD, Susan Gussenhoven, PhD, John Shaw, MS, Michael Squillante, PhD, Kevin Buckley, CHP, Jayne Caruso, Victor Lee, MD, Toby Wroblicka, MD, Dan Winder, MD, Dennis Atkinson, MD, and Inna Gazit, MD. Thanks to Peter Shomphe, ARRT, CNMT, Bob Dann, PhD, and Laura Partriquin, MD, for wading through the manuscript in its entirety. We greatly appreciate the patience shown at that time by Robert Zimmerman, MSEE, Kevin Buckley, CHP, John Widman, PhD, CHP, Peter Waer, PhD, Stephen Moore, PhD, Bill Worstell, PhD, and Hernan Jara, PhD, while answering our numerous questions. Thanks to Delia Edwards, Milda Pitter, and Paul Guidone, MD, for taking time to pose as models. The authors would also like to thank Rhoda M. Powsner, MD, for her assistance in reviewing sections of the text and for proofreading the review questions.

CHAPTER 1

Basic Nuclear Medicine Physics

Properties and structure of matter

Matter has several fundamental properties. For our purposes, the most important are mass and charge (electric). We recognize mass by the force gravity exerts on a material object (commonly referred to as its weight) and by the object's inertia, which is the "resistance" we encounter when we attempt to change the position or motion of a material object.

Similarly, we can, at least at times, recognize charge by the direct effect it can have on us or that we can observe it to have on inanimate objects. For example, we may feel the presence of a strongly charged object when it causes our hair to move or even to stand on end. More often than not, however, we are insensitive to charge. But whether grossly detectable or not, its effects must be considered here because of the role charge plays in the structure of matter.

Charge is generally thought to have been recognized first by the ancient Greeks. They noticed that some kinds of matter, an amber rod for example, can be given an electric charge by rubbing it with a piece of cloth. Their experiments convinced them that there are two kinds of charge: opposite charges, which attract each other, and like charges, which repel. One kind of charge came to be called positive, and the other negative. We now know that negative charge is associated with electrons. The rubbing transferred some of the electrons from the atoms of the matter in the rod to the cloth. In a similar fashion, electrons can be transferred from a cat's fur to a hand. After petting, the cat will have a net positive charge and the person a net negative charge

(Figure 1.1). With these basic properties in mind, we can look at matter in more detail.

Matter is composed of molecules. In any chemically pure material, the molecules are the smallest units that retain the characteristics of the material itself. For example, if a block of salt were to be broken into successively smaller pieces, the smallest fragment with the properties of salt would be a single salt molecule (Figure 1.2). With further fragmentation, the molecule would no longer be salt. Molecules, in turn, are composed of atoms. Most molecules consist of more than one kind of atom—salt, for example, is made up of atoms of chlorine and atoms of sodium. The atoms themselves are composed of smaller particles, the subatomic particles, which are discussed later. The molecule is held together by chemical bonds among its atoms. These bonds are formed by the force of electrical attraction between oppositely charged parts of the molecule. This force is often referred to as the Coulomb force after Charles A. de Coulomb, the physicist who characterized it. This is the force involved in chemical reactions such as the combining of hydrogen and oxygen to form water. The electrons of the atom are held by the electrical force between them and the positive nucleus. The nucleus of the atom is held together by another type of force—the nuclear force—which is involved in the release of atomic energy. Nuclear forces are orders of magnitude greater than electrical forces.

Elements

There are more than 100 species of atoms. These species are referred to as elements. Most of the

---

Essentials of Nuclear Medicine Physics and Instrumentation, Third Edition. Rachel A. Powsner, Matthew R. Palmer, and Edward R. Powsner.
© 2013 John Wiley & Sons, Ltd. Published 2013 by John Wiley & Sons, Ltd.

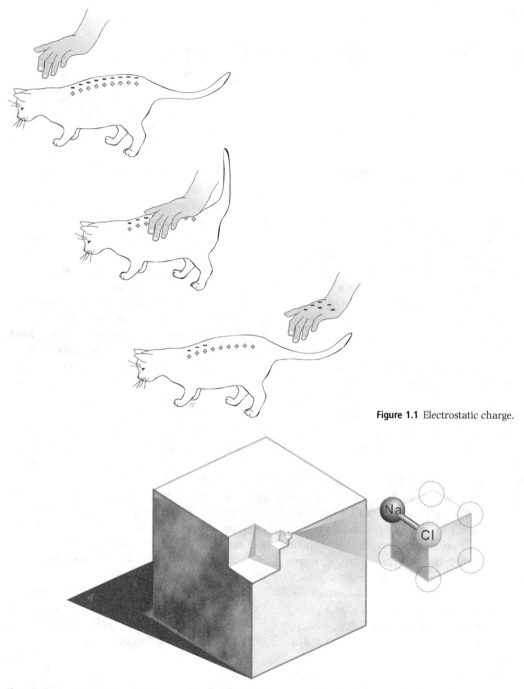

Figure 1.1 Electrostatic charge.

Figure 1.2 The NaCl molecule is the smallest unit of salt that retains the characteristics of salt.

known elements—for example, mercury, helium, gold, hydrogen, and oxygen—occur naturally on earth; others are not usually found in nature but are made by humans—for example, europium and americium. A reasonable explanation for the absence of some elements from nature is that if and when they were formed, they proved too unstable to survive in detectable amounts into the present.

All the elements have been assigned symbols or abbreviated chemical names, for example gold, Au; mercury, Hg; and helium, He. Some symbols are obvious abbreviations of the English name; others

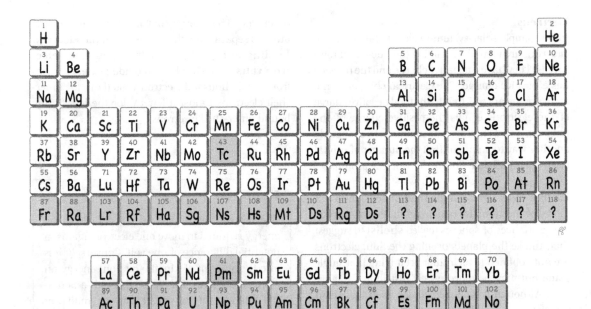

Figure 1.3 Periodic table.

are derived from the original Latin name of the element. For example, Au is from *aurum*, the Latin word for gold.

All of the known elements, both natural and those made by humans, can be organized into the **periodic table**. In Figure 1.3, the elements that have a stable state are shown in white boxes; those that occur only in a radioactive form are shown in gray boxes. The number appearing above each element's abbreviation is referred to as the atomic number, which will be discussed later in this chapter.

The elements in the periodic table are arranged in columns (called groups) and rows (called periods). In general, elements within groups demonstrate similar properties. This is because elements in a group often have similar numbers of electrons in their outer shell; outer-shell electron configurations are more important in determining how an atom interacts with other elemental atoms. The lanthanides and actinides are special groups of elements, conventionally shown in rows separated from and placed below the table. These two groups have the same number of outer-shell electrons and share many common properties.

Atomic structure

Atoms initially were thought of as no more than small pieces of matter. Our understanding that they

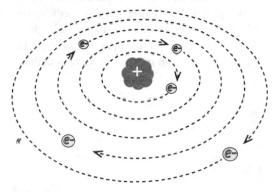

Figure 1.4 Flat atom. The standard two-dimensional drawing of atomic structure.

have an inner structure has its roots in the observations of earlier physicists that the atoms of which matter is composed contain **electrons** of negative charge. Inasmuch as the atom as a whole is electrically neutral, it seemed obvious that it must also contain something with a positive charge to balance the negative charge of the electrons. Thus, early attempts to picture the atom, modeled on our solar system, showed the negatively charged electrons orbiting a central group of particles, the positively charged **nucleus** (Figure 1.4).

Electrons

In our simple solar-system model of the atom, the electrons are viewed as orbiting the nucleus at high speeds. They have a negative charge and the nucleus has a positive charge. The electrical charges of the atom are "balanced," that is, the total negative charge of the electrons equals the positive charge of the nucleus. As we shall see in a moment, this is simply another way to point out that the number of orbital electrons equals the number of nuclear protons.

Electron shells: By adding a third dimension to our model of the atom, we can depict the electron orbits as the surfaces of spheres (called **shells**) to suggest that, unlike the planets orbiting the Sun, electrons are not confined to a circular orbit lying in a single plane but may be more widely distributed (Figure 1.5). Although it is convenient for us to talk about the distances and diameters of the shells, distance on the atomic scale does not have quite the same meaning as it does with everyday objects. The more significant characteristic of a shell is the energy that it signifies. The "closer" an electron is to the nucleus, the more tightly it is bound to the nucleus. In saying this, we mean that more work (energy) is required to remove an inner-shell electron than an outer one. The energy that must be put into the atom to separate an electron is called the **electron binding energy**. It is usually expressed in **electron volts** (eV). The electron binding energy varies from a few thousand electron volts (keV) for inner-shell electrons to just a few eV for the less tightly bound outer-shell electrons.

Electron volt

The electron volt is a special unit defined as the energy required to move one electron against a potential difference of one volt. Conversely, it is also the amount of kinetic (motion) energy an electron acquires if it "falls" through a potential difference of one volt. It is a very small unit on the everyday scale, at only 1.6×10^{-19} joules (J), but a very convenient unit on the atomic scale. The joule is the Système International (SI) unit of work or energy. For comparison, 1 J equals 0.24 small calories (as opposed to the large calorie (kcal) used to measure food intake).

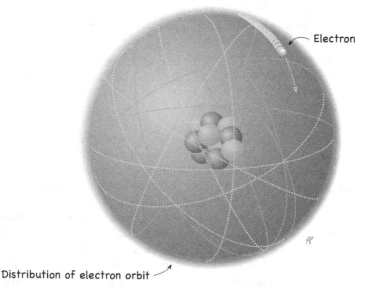

Electron

Distribution of electron orbit

Figure 1.5 An electron shell is a representation of the energy level associated with an atomic electron.

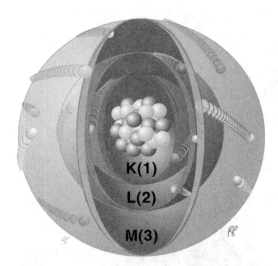

Figure 1.6 K, L, and M electron shells.

Quantum numbers: The atomic electrons in their shells are usually described by their quantum numbers, of which there are four types. The first is the **principal quantum number** (n), which identifies the energy shell. The first three shells (K, L, and M) are depicted in Figure 1.6. The electron binding energy is greatest for the innermost shell (K) and is progressively less for the outer shells. Larger atoms have more shells.

The second (azimuthal), third (magnetic), and fourth (spin) quantum numbers refer to other physical properties of the electron. Each electron within an atom has a unique combination of the four quantum numbers.

The maximum number of electrons associated with each energy shell is $2n^2$, where n is the shell number. The first shell (the K shell) can contain a maximum of two electrons, the second shell (the L shell) can contain a maximum of eight electrons, the third shell (the M shell) can contain a maximum of 18 electrons, and so on.

Representation of electron distribution: Most of the diagrams (for example Figure 1.6) in this chapter reflect what is referred to as the **Bohr model** of the atom and, as such, all electrons within each shell are depicted as moving along the surface of a sphere, each shell represented as one such sphere with a distinct radial distance from a centrally located nucleus. The radius of these spheres increases with the principal quantum number. This

model of the atom is frequently used for teaching purposes because the radial distance of an electron from the nucleus is used to depict how tightly bound it is to the atom—the closest electrons being most tightly bound.

A more accurate quantum mechanical description of the electron distribution uses a sequence of **orbitals**. Orbitals are mathematical functions that describe the probability of finding an electron in a region of space near the nucleus. For each principal quantum number (each shell), there is a spherical orbital, denoted by the principal quantum number followed by the letter "s." This orbital contains two electrons (Figure 1.7(a)). This is the only orbital for the K shell, which contains at maximum two electrons, and this orbital is called the **1s orbital**. The neutral atom with a full K shell is the helium atom.

The next shell, the L shell ($n = 2$), also has a spherical orbital, denoted 2s (also depicted in Figure 1.7(a)), which contains two electrons, as well as three suborbitals, denoted $2p_x$, $2p_y$, $2p_z$. Each suborbital has a shape like a dumbbell or a three-dimensional figure of eight (see Figure 1.7(b)). The three suborbitals are oriented along three orthogonal axes, as shown in Figure 1.7(c). Each suborbital is filled by two electrons; the neutral atom with completely filled orbitals for $n = 1$ and $n = 2$ is neon. For the higher-order orbitals, with $n > 2$, the suborbitals associated with higher azimuthal quantum numbers become even more complicated in structure and will not be discussed here.

Quantum numbers

The term **quantum** means literally "amount." It acquired its special significance in physics when Bohr and others theorized that physical quantities such as energy and light could not have a range of values as on a continuum, but rather could have only discrete, step-like values. The individual steps are so small that their existence escaped the notice of physicists until Bohr postulated them to explain his theory of the atom. We now refer to Bohr's theory as **quantum theory**, and the resulting explanations of motion on the atomic scale as **quantum mechanics** to distinguish it from the classical mechanics described by Isaac Newton, which is still needed for everyday engineering.

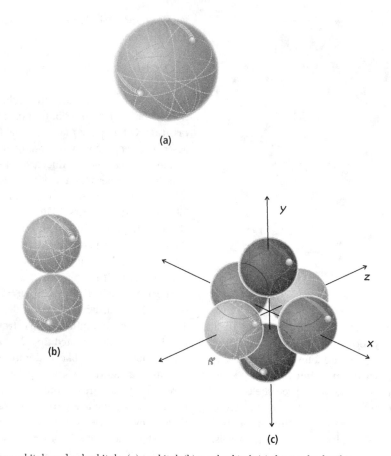

Figure 1.7 Electron orbitals and suborbitals. (a) s orbital; (b) p suborbital; (c) the p suborbitals p_x, p_y, p_z.

Stable electron configuration: Just as it takes energy to remove an electron from its atom, it takes energy to move an electron from an inner shell to an outer shell, which can also be thought of as the energy required to pull a negative electron away from the positively charged nucleus. Any vacancy in an inner shell creates an unstable condition, often referred to as an **excited state**.

The electrical charges of the atom are balanced, that is, the total negative charge of the electrons equals the total positive charge of the nucleus. This is simply another way of pointing out that the number of orbital electrons equals the number of nuclear protons. Furthermore, the electrons must fill the shells with the highest binding energy first. At least in the elements of low-atomic-number electrons, the inner shells have the highest binding energy.

If the arrangement of the electrons in the shells is not in the stable state, they will undergo rearrangement in order to become stable, a process often referred to as **de-excitation**. Because the stable configuration of the shells always has less energy than any unstable configuration, the de-excitation releases energy as photons, often as **X-rays**.

Nucleus
Like the atom itself, the atomic nucleus also has an inner structure (Figure 1.8). Experiments have shown that the nucleus consists of two types of particles: **protons**, which carry a positive charge, and **neutrons**, which carry no charge. The general term for protons and neutrons is **nucleons**. The nucleons, as shown in the first two rows of Table 1.1, have a much greater mass than electrons. Like

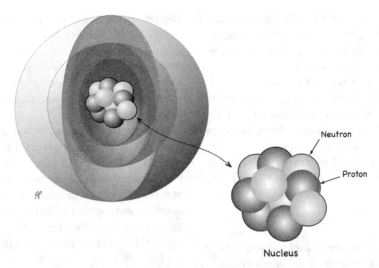

Figure 1.8 The nucleus of an atom is composed of protons and neutrons.

Table 1.1 The subatomic particles

Name	Symbol	Location	Mass[a]	Charge
Neutron	n	Nucleus	1839	None
Proton	p	Nucleus	1836	Positive (+)
Electron	e⁻	Shell	1	Negative (−)

[a]Relative to an electron.

electrons, nucleons have quantum properties, including spin. The nucleus has a spin value equal to the sum of the nucleon spin values.

A simple but useful model of the nucleus is a tightly bound cluster of protons and neutrons. Protons naturally repel each other, since they are positively charged; however, there is a powerful binding force called the **nuclear force** that holds the nucleons together very tightly (Figure 1.9). The work (energy) required to overcome the nuclear force, the work to remove a nucleon from the nucleus, is called the **nuclear binding energy**. Typical binding energies are in the range of 6 million to 9 million electron volts (MeV) (approximately one thousand to one million times the electron binding force). The magnitude of the binding energy is related to another fact of nature: the measured mass of a nucleus is always less than the mass expected from the sum of the masses of its neutrons and protons. The "missing" mass is called the **mass defect**, the energy equivalent of which is

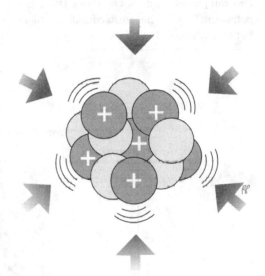

Figure 1.9 The nuclear binding force is strong enough to overcome the electrical repulsion between the positively charged protons.

equal to the nuclear binding energy. This interchangeability of mass and energy was immortalized in Einstein's equation $E = mc^2$.

The stable nucleus: Not all elements have stable nuclei; however, they do exist for most of the light and mid-weight elements, i.e., those with **atomic numbers** (number of protons) up to and including bismuth ($Z = 83$). The exceptions are technetium

($Z = 43$) and promethium ($Z = 61$). All those with atomic numbers higher than 83, such as radium ($Z = 88$) and uranium ($Z = 92$), are inherently unstable because of their large size.

For those nuclei with a stable state, there is an optimal ratio of neutrons to protons. For the lighter elements, this ratio is approximately 1:1; for increasing atomic weights, the number of neutrons exceeds the number of protons. A plot depicting the number of neutrons as a function of the number of protons is called the **line of stability** (Figure 1.10).

Stability

Strictly speaking, stability is a relative term. We call a nuclide stable when its half-life is so long as to be practically immeasurable—say, greater than 10^8 years. The isotope of potassium ^{40}K, for example, which makes up about 1% of the potassium found in nature, is considered stable but actually has a half-life of 10^9 years.

Isotopes, isotones, and isobars: Each atom of any sample of an element has the same number of protons (the same Z, i.e., atomic number) in its nucleus. Lead found anywhere in the world will always be composed of atoms with 82 protons. The same does not apply, however, to the number of neutrons in the nucleus.

An **isotope** of an element is a particular variation of the nuclear composition of the atoms of that element. The number of protons (Z) is unchanged, but the number of neutrons (N) varies. Since the number of neutrons changes, the total number of neutrons and protons (A, the atomic mass) changes. The chemical symbol for each element can be expanded to include these three numbers (Figure 1.11).

Two related entities are **isotones** and **isobars**. Isotones are atoms of different elements that contain identical numbers of neutrons but varying numbers of protons. Isobars are atoms of different elements with identical numbers of nucleons. Examples of these are illustrated in Figure 1.12.

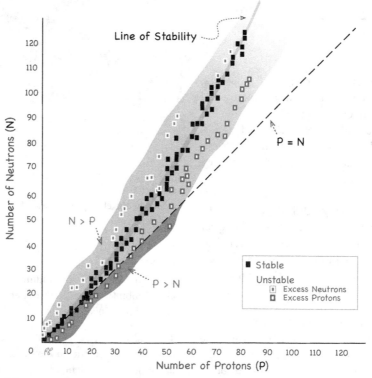

Figure 1.10 The combinations of neutrons and protons that can coexist in a stable nuclear configuration all lie within the gray-shaded regions.

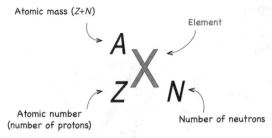

Figure 1.11 Standard atomic notation.

Radioactivity

The unstable nucleus and radioactive decay

A nucleus not in its stable state will adjust itself until it is more stable either by ejecting portions of its nucleus or by emitting energy in the form of photons (gamma rays). This process is referred to as radioactive decay. The type of decay depends on which of the following rules for nuclear stability is violated.

Excessive nuclear mass

Alpha decay: Very large unstable atoms, atoms with high atomic mass, may split into nuclear fragments. The smallest stable nuclear fragment that is emitted is a particle consisting of two neutrons and two protons, equivalent to the nucleus of a helium atom. Because it was one of the first types of radiation discovered, the emission of a helium nucleus is called **alpha radiation**, and the emitted helium nucleus an **alpha particle** (Figure 1.13).

Fission: Under some circumstances, the nucleus of an unstable atom may break into larger fragments, a process usually referred to as **nuclear fission**. During fission, two or three neutrons are emitted (Figure 1.14).

Unstable neutron–proton ratio

Too many neutrons: beta decay: Nuclei with excess neutrons can achieve stability by a process that amounts to the conversion of a neutron into a proton and an electron. The proton remains in the nucleus, but the electron is emitted. This is called **beta radiation**, and the electron itself a **beta particle** (Figure 1.15). The process and the emitted

electron were given these names to contrast with the alpha particle before the physical nature of either was discovered. The beta particle generated in this decay will become a free electron until it finds a vacancy in an electron shell in another atom.

Careful study of beta decay suggested to physicists that the conversion of a neutron to a proton involved more than the emission of a beta particle (electron). Beta emission satisfied the rule for conservation of charge in that the neutral neutron yielded one positive proton and one negative electron; however, it did not appear to satisfy the equally important rule for conservation of energy. Measurements showed that most of the emitted electrons simply did not have all the energy expected. To explain this apparent discrepancy, the emission of a second particle was postulated, and that particle was later identified experimentally. Called an **antineutrino** (the "neutrino" is for "small and neutral"), it carries the "missing" energy of the reaction.

Too many protons: positron decay and electron capture: In a manner analogous to that for excess neutrons, an unstable nucleus with too many protons can undergo a decay that has the effect of converting a proton into a neutron. There are two ways this can occur: positron decay and electron capture. In general, proton-rich nuclei decay by a combination of these two processes.

Positron decay: A proton can be converted into a neutron and a **positron**, which is an electron with a positive, instead of negative, charge (Figure 1.16). The positron is also referred to as a positive beta particle, positive electron, or antielectron. In positron decay, a **neutrino** is also emitted. In many ways, positron decay is the mirror image of beta decay: positive electron instead of negative electron, neutrino instead of antineutrino. Unlike the negative electron, the positron itself survives only briefly. It quickly encounters an electron (electrons are plentiful in matter), and both are **annihilated** (see Chapter 8, Figure 8.1). This is why it is considered an antielectron. Generally speaking, antiparticles react with the corresponding particle to annihilate both.

During the annihilation reaction, the combined mass of the positron and electron is converted into two photons of energy equivalent to the mass

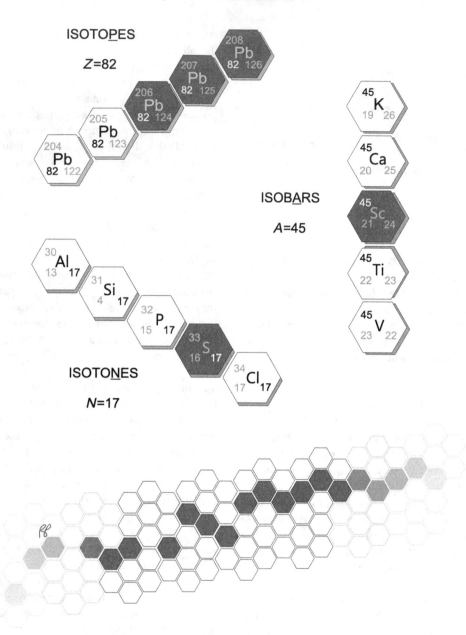

Figure 1.12 Nuclides of the same atomic number but different atomic mass are called isotopes, those of an equal number of neutrons are called isotones, and those of the same atomic mass but different atomic number are called isobars. Stable nuclear configurations are shaded gray, and radioactive configurations are white. (Adapted from Brucer, M., *Trilinear Chart of the Nuclides*, Mallinckrodt Inc., 1979.)

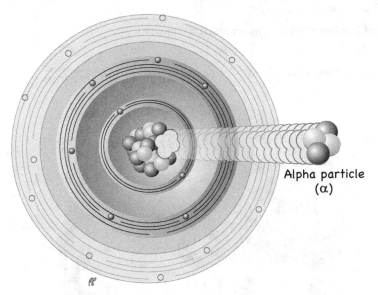

Alpha particle
(α)

Figure 1.13 Alpha decay.

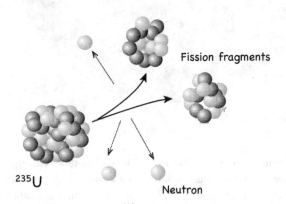

Fission fragments

^{235}U

Neutron

Figure 1.14 Fission of a ^{235}U nucleus.

Antineutrino $\overline{\nu}$

Beta particle (β⁻)

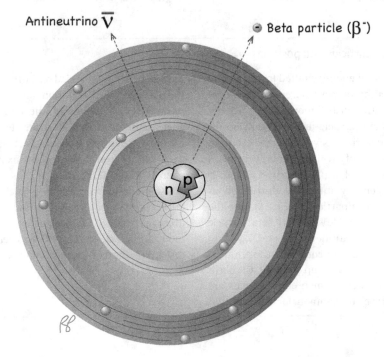

Figure 1.15 β⁻ (negatron) decay.

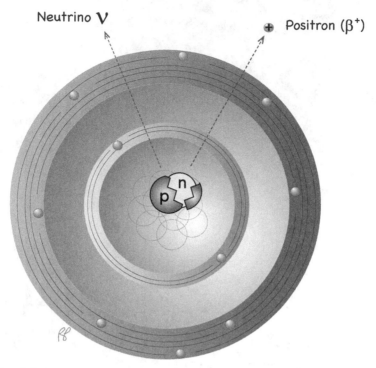

Figure 1.16 β^+ (positron) decay.

destroyed. Unless the difference between the masses of the parent and daughter atoms is at least equal to the mass of one electron plus one positron, a total equivalent to 1.02 MeV, there will be insufficient energy available for positron emission.

Electron capture: Through a process that competes with positron decay, a nucleus can combine with one of its inner orbital electrons to achieve the net effect of converting one of the protons in the nucleus into a neutron (Figure 1.18). An outer-

---

Energy of beta particles and positrons

Although the total energy emitted from an atom during beta decay or positron emission is constant, the relative distribution of this energy between the beta particle and antineutrino (or positron and neutrino) is variable. For example, the total amount of available energy released during beta decay of a phosphorus-32 atom is 1.7 MeV. This energy might be distributed as 0.5 MeV to the beta particle and 1.2 MeV to the antineutrino, or 1.5 MeV to the beta particle and 0.2 MeV to the antineutrino, or 1.7 MeV to the beta particle and no energy to the antineutrino, and so on. In any group of atoms, the likelihoods of occurrence of such combinations are not equal. It is very uncommon, for example, that

all of the energy is carried off by the beta particle. It is much more common for the particle to receive less than half of the total amount of energy emitted. This is illustrated by Figure 1.17, a plot of the number of beta particles emitted at each energy from zero to the maximum energy released in the decay. Here, $E_{\beta\,max}$ is the maximum possible energy that a beta particle can receive during beta decay of any atom, and $\overline{E}_\beta$ is the average energy of all beta particles for decay of a group of such atoms. The average energy is approximately one-third of the maximum energy, or

$$\overline{E}_\beta \cong \frac{1}{3} E_{\beta\,max}$$

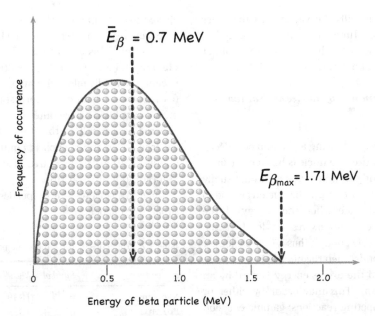

Figure 1.17 Beta emissions (both β⁻ and β⁺) are ejected from the nucleus with energies between 0 and their maximum possible energy ($E_{\beta\,max}$). The average energy ($\bar{E}_\beta$) is equal to approximately one-third of the maximum energy.

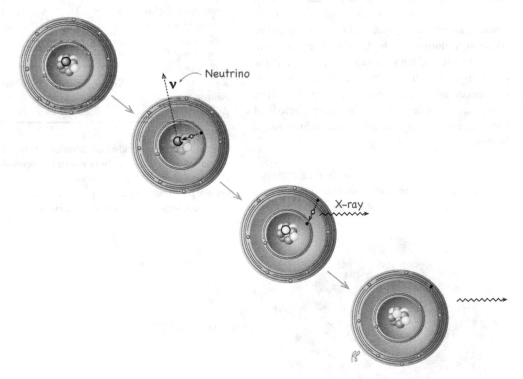

Figure 1.18 Electron capture.

shell electron then fills the vacancy in the inner shell left by the captured electron. The energy lost by the "fall" of the outer-shell electron to the inner shell is emitted as an X-ray.

Appropriate numbers of nucleons, but too much energy

Isomeric transition: Following alpha and beta decay and electron capture, the nucleus has a more favorable physical configuration of nucleons but usually contains an excess of energy. The nucleus is said to be in an excited state when the energy of the nucleus is greater than its resting level. If the excited state is stable enough (has a half-life longer than 10–12 seconds) then the nuclide is referred to as an isomer and the excess energy is shed by an isomeric transition. This may occur by either or both of two competing reactions: gamma emission and internal conversion. Most isomeric transitions occur as a combination of these two reactions.

Gamma emission: In this process, excess nuclear energy is emitted as a gamma ray (Figure 1.19). The name "gamma" was given to this radiation, before its physical nature was understood, because it was the third (alpha, beta, gamma) type of radiation discovered. A gamma ray is a photon (energy) emitted by an excited nucleus. Despite its unique name, it cannot be distinguished from photons of the same energy from a different source, for example X-rays.

Internal conversion: The excited nucleus can transfer its excess energy to an orbital electron (generally an inner-shell electron), causing the electron to be ejected from the atom. This can only occur if the excess energy is greater than the binding energy of the electron. This electron is called a **conversion electron** (Figure 1.20). The resulting inner-orbital vacancy is rapidly filled with an outer-shell electron (as the atom assumes a more stable state, inner orbitals are filled before outer orbitals). The energy released as a result of the "fall" of an outer-shell electron to an inner shell is emitted as an X-ray (Figure 1.20(a)) or as a free electron, an **Auger electron** (Figure 1.20(b)).

Table 1.2 reviews the properties of the various subatomic particles.

Table 1.2 Properties of the subatomic particles

Name(s)	Symbol	Mass[a]	Charge
Neutron	n	1839	None
Proton	p	1836	Positive (+)
Electron	e^-	1	Negative (−)
Beta particle (beta-minus particle, electron)[b]	β^-	1	Negative (−)
Positron (beta-plus particle, positive electron)	β^+	1	Positive (+)
Gamma ray (photon)	γ	None	None
X-ray	X-ray	None	None
Neutrino	ν	Near zero	None
Antineutrino	$\bar{\nu}$	Near zero	None

[a]Relative to an electron.
[b]There is no physical difference between a beta particle and an electron; the term **beta particle** is applied to an electron that is emitted from a radioactive nucleus. The symbol β without a minus or plus sign attached always refers to a beta-minus particle, or electron.

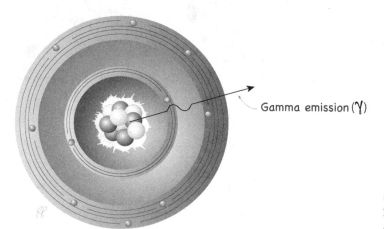

Figure 1.19 Isomeric transition. Excess nuclear energy is carried off as a gamma ray.

Gamma emission (γ)

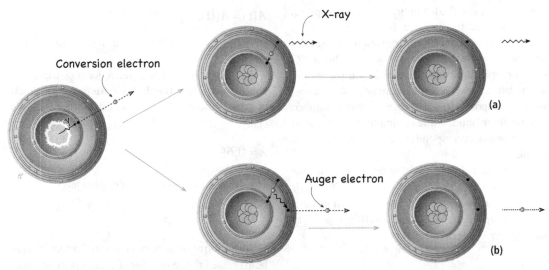

Figure 1.20 Internal conversion. As an alternative to gamma emission, it can lead to emission of either an X-ray (a) or an Auger electron (b).

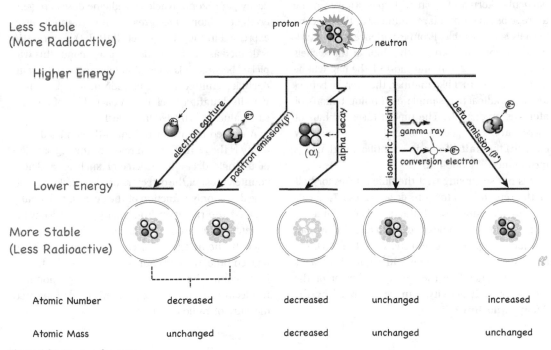

		decreased	decreased	unchanged	increased
Atomic Number		decreased	decreased	unchanged	increased
Atomic Mass		unchanged	decreased	unchanged	unchanged

Figure 1.21 Decay schematics.

Decay notation

Decay from an unstable parent nuclide to a more stable daughter nuclide can occur in a series of steps, with the production of particles and photons characteristic of each step. A standard notation is used to describe these steps (Figure 1.21). The uppermost level of the schematic is the state with the greatest energy. As the nuclide decays by losing energy and/or particles, lower horizontal levels represent states of relatively lower energy. Directional arrows from one level to the next indicate the type of decay. By convention, an oblique line angled downward and to the left indicates electron capture; downward and to the right, beta emission; and a vertical arrow, an isomeric transition. A dogleg is used for positron emission. A dogleg with a "Z" denotes alpha decay. Notice that a pathway ending to the left, as in electron capture or positron emission, corresponds to a decrease in atomic number. On the other hand, a line ending to the right, as in beta emission, corresponds to an increase in atomic number.

Figure 1.22 depicts specific decay schemes for ^{99m}Tc, ^{111}In, ^{131}I, and ^{226}Ra. The "m" in ^{99m}Tc stands for **metastable**, which refers to an excited nucleus with an appreciable lifetime ($>10^{-12}$ s) prior to undergoing isomeric transition.

Half-life

It is not possible to predict when an individual nuclide atom will decay, just as in preparing popcorn, where one cannot determine when any particular kernel of corn will open. However, the average behavior of a large number of the popcorn kernels is predictable. From experience with microwave popcorn, one knows that half of the kernels will pop within 2 min and most of the bag will be done in 4 min. In a like manner, the average behavior of a radioactive sample containing billions of atoms is predictable. The time it takes for half of these atoms to decay is called (appropriately enough) the **half-life** or, in scientific notation, $T_{1/2}$ (pronounced "T one-half").

It is not surprising that the time it takes for half of the remaining atoms to decay is also $T_{1/2}$. This process continues until the number of nuclide atoms eventually comes so close to zero that we can consider the process complete. A plot of $A(t)$, the activity remaining, is shown in Figure 1.23. This curve, and therefore the average behavior of the sample of radioactivity, can be described by the **decay equation**,

$$A(t) = A(0)e^{-0.693t/T_{1/2}}$$

where $A(0)$ is the initial number of radioactive atoms.

A commonly used alternative form of the decay equation employs the **decay constant** (λ), which is approximately 0.693 divided by the half-life ($T_{1/2}$):

$$\lambda = 0.693/T_{1/2}$$

The decay equation can be rewritten as

$$A(t) = A(0)e^{-\lambda t}$$

The amount of activity of any radionuclide may be expressed as the number of decays per unit time. Common units for measuring radioactivity are the **curie** (after Marie Curie) and the SI unit, the **becquerel** (after another nuclear pioneer, Henri Becquerel). One becquerel is defined as one radioactive decay per second. Nuclear medicine doses are generally a million times greater and are more easily expressed in megabecquerels (MBq). One curie (Ci) is defined as 3.7×10^{10} decays per second (this was picked because it is approximately equal to the radioactivity emitted by 1 g of radium in equilibrium with its daughter nuclides). A partial list of conversion values is provided in Table 1.3.

A related term that is frequently confused with decay is the **count**, which refers to the registration of a single decay by a detector such as a Geiger counter. Most of the detectors used in nuclear medicine detect only a fraction of the decays, principally because the radiation from many of the decays is directed away from the detector. The count rate refers to the number of decays actually counted in a given time, usually counts per minute. All things being equal, the count rate will be proportional to the decay rate, and it is a commonly used, if inexact, measure of radioactivity.

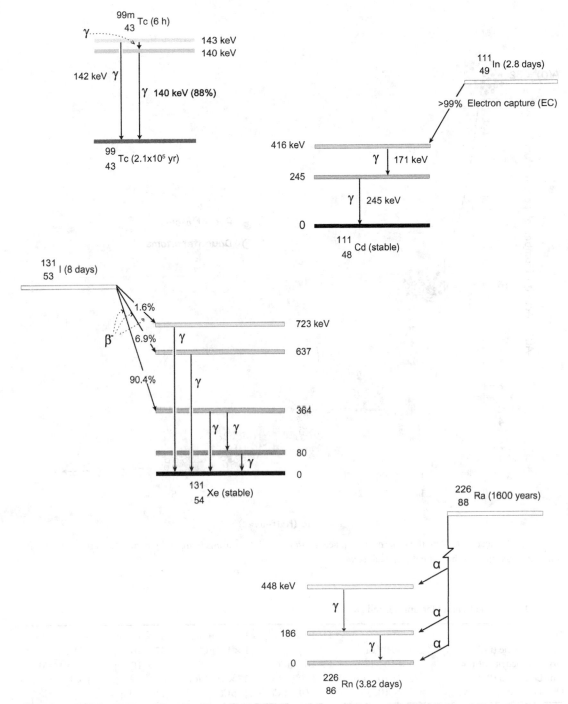

Figure 1.22 Decay schemes showing principal transitions for technetium-99m, indium-111, iodine-131, and radium-226. Energy levels are rounded to three significant figures.

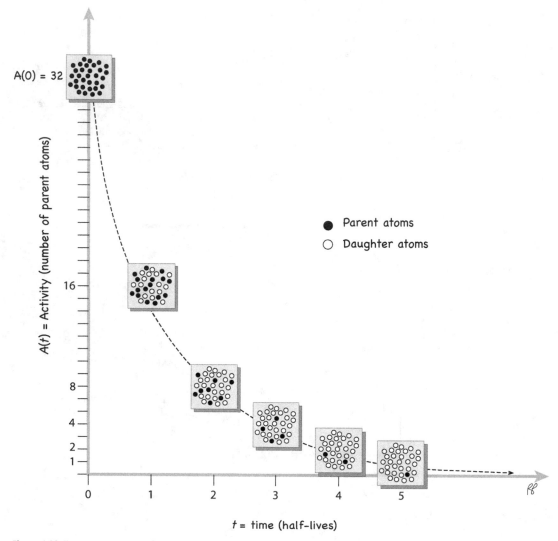

Figure 1.23 Decay curve. Note the progressive replacement of radioactive atoms (parent) by relatively more stable atoms (daughter) as shown schematically in each box.

Table 1.3 Conversion values for units of radioactivity

One curie (Ci) =		1×10^3 mCi	1×10^6 µCi	37×10^9 Bq	37×10^3 MBq
One millicurie (mCi) =	1×10^{-3} Ci		1×10^3 µCi	37×10^6 Bq	37 MBq
One microcurie (µCi) =	1×10^{-6} Ci	1×10^{-3} mCi		37×10^3 Bq	37×10^{-3} MBq
One becquerel (Bq)[a] =	27×10^{-12} Ci	27×10^{-9} mCi	27×10^{-6} µCi		1×10^{-6} MBq
One megabecquerel (MBq) =	27×10^{-6} Ci	27×10^{-3} mCi	27 µCi	1×10^6 Bq	

[a]One becquerel = 1 decay per second.

Questions

1. The chemical interactions between various elements are mainly determined by:
   (a) The number of protons.
   (b) The number of neutrons.
   (c) The number of electrons in the outermost shell.
   (d) The number of protons minus the number of electrons.

2. For each of the five terms below, choose the best definition:
   (1) Isobars.
   (2) Isoclines.
   (3) Isomers.
   (4) Isotones.
   (5) Isotopes.
   (a) Atoms of the same element (equal Z) with different numbers of neutrons (N).
   (b) Atoms of the same element (equal Z) with different numbers of protons.
   (c) Atoms of different elements (different Z) with equal numbers of neutrons (N).
   (d) Atoms of different elements with equal atomic mass (A).

3. Which of the following statements are correct?
   (a) There is a stable isotope of technetium.
   (b) Atoms with atomic numbers $Z > 83$ are inherently unstable.
   (c) For light elements, nuclear stability is achieved with equal numbers of protons and neutrons; for heavier elements, the number of neutrons exceeds the number of protons.

4. For internal conversion to occur, the excess energy of the excited nucleus must equal or exceed:
   (a) $0.551\,eV$.
   (b) $1.102\,eV$.
   (c) The internal conversion coefficient.
   (d) The average energy of the Auger electrons.
   (e) The binding energy of the emitted electron.

5. For an atom undergoing beta decay, the average energy of the emitted beta particles is approximately:
   (a) $0.551\,eV$.
   (b) 0.551 times the loss of atomic mass.

(c) One-half of the total energy released for the individual event.
   (d) One-third of the maximum energy of the emitted beta particles.
   (e) The average energy of the accompanying antineutrinos.

6. You receive a dose of ^{99m}Tc measuring $370\,MBq$ from the radiopharmacy at $10\,AM$. Your patient does not arrive in the department until $2\,PM$. How much activity, in mCi, remains? (The $T_{1/2}$ of ^{99m}Tc is $6\,h$. The constant e is equal to 2.718.)

7. Rank the following binding energies from largest to smallest:
   (1) Electron binding energy for outer-shell electrons.
   (2) Nuclear binding energy.
   (3) Electron binding energy for inner-shell electrons.

8. True or false: The term "metastable" refers to an intermediate state of nuclear decay lasting longer than $10^{-12}\,s$ prior to undergoing isomeric transition.

9. Which of the following is true regarding beta decay of a specific radioisotope?
   (1) The energy of the emitted beta particle is always the same.
   (2) The energy of the emitted antineutrino is always the same.
   (3) The summed energy of the emitted beta particle and antineutrino is always the same.

10. Which unit of measurement for radioactivity is defined as one radioactive decay per second?
    (1) Becquerel.
    (2) Millicurie.
    (3) Megabecquerel

11. $10\,mCi$ equals how many MBq?
    (1) $2.7\,MBq$.
    (2) $37\,MBq$.
    (3) $270\,MBq$.
    (4) $370\,MBq$.

12. Lighter nuclides $(Z < 83)$ with an excess of neutrons tend to decay by
    (1) Gamma emission.
    (2) Beta-minus decay.

(3) Isomeric transition.

(4) Positron emission.

(5) Alpha emission.

13. Which of the following statements are true?

(1) An alpha particle is the same thing as a helium nucleus.

(2) Neutrinos have the same charge as an electron.

(3) X-rays always have lower energies than gamma rays.

(4) The terms "activity" and "count rate" are the same—they express a measurement of photons per second.

14. When orbital electrons move from an outer shell to an inner shell, which of the following is **not** true?

(a) Characteristic X-rays can be emitted.

(b) Auger electrons can be emitted.

(c) The atom becomes more stable.

(d) A mixture of gamma rays and internal conversion electrons can be emitted.

(e) The atom is still in an ionized state.

Answers

1. (c).

2. (1) (d). (2) None of the above; usually used as a geological term. (3) None of the above; in nuclear medicine, it refers to an element whose nucleus is in an unstable (excited) state. (4) (c). (5) (a).

3. (b) and (c) are true. (a) is false: technetium does not have a stable form. ^{99}Tc has a $T_{1/2}$ of 2.1×10^5 yr.

4. (e).

5. (d).

6. 6.3 mCi.

7. Nuclear binding energy, electron binding energy for inner-shell electrons, electron binding energy for outer-shell electrons.

8. True.

9. (3).

10. Becquerel.

11. 370 MBq.

12. (2).

13. (1) only.

14. (d).

CHAPTER 2

Interaction of Radiation with Matter

When radiation strikes matter, both the nature of the radiation and the composition of the matter affect what happens. The process begins with the transfer of radiation energy to the atoms and molecules, heating the matter or even modifying its structure.

If all the energy of a bombarding particle or photon is transferred, the radiation will appear to have been stopped within the irradiated matter. Conversely, if the energy is not completely deposited in the matter, the remaining energy will emerge as though the matter were transparent or at least translucent. This said, we shall now introduce some of the physical phenomena that are involved as radiation interacts with matter, and in particular we shall consider, separately at first, the interactions in matter of both photons (gamma rays and X-rays) and charged particles (alpha and beta particles).

Interaction of photons with matter

As they pass through matter, photons interact with atoms. The type of interaction is a function of the energy of the photons and the atomic number (Z) of the elements composing the matter.

Types of photon interactions in matter

In the practice of nuclear medicine, where gamma rays with energies between 50 and 550 keV are used, **Compton scattering** is the dominant type of interaction in materials with lower atomic numbers, such as human tissue (Z = 7.5). The **photoelectric effect** is the dominant type of interaction in materials with higher atomic numbers, such as lead (Z = 82). A third type of interaction of photons with matter, **pair production**, only occurs with very high photon energies (greater than 1020 keV) and is therefore not important in clinical nuclear medicine. Figure 2.1 depicts the predominant types of interaction for various combinations of incident photons and absorber atomic numbers.

Compton scattering

In Compton scattering, the incident photon transfers part of its energy to an outer-shell or (essentially) "free" electron, ejecting it from the atom. Upon ejection, this electron is called a **Compton electron**. The photon, which has lost energy in the interaction, is scattered (Figure 2.2) at an angle that depends on the amount of energy transferred from the photon to the electron. The scattering angle can range from nearly 0° to 180°. Figure 2.3 illustrates scattering angles of 135° and 45°.

Photoelectric effect

An incident photon may also transfer its energy to an orbital (generally inner-shell) electron. This process is called the photoelectric effect and the ejected electron is called a **photoelectron** (Figure 2.4). This electron leaves the atom with an energy equal to the energy of the incident gamma ray diminished by the binding energy of the electron. An outer-shell electron then fills the inner-shell vacancy, and the excess energy is emitted as an X-ray:

$$E_{photoelectron} = E_{photon} - E_{binding}$$

Table 2.1 lists the predominant photon interactions in some common materials.

Essentials of Nuclear Medicine Physics and Instrumentation, Third Edition. Rachel A. Powsner, Matthew R. Palmer, and Edward R. Powsner.
© 2013 John Wiley & Sons, Ltd. Published 2013 by John Wiley & Sons, Ltd.

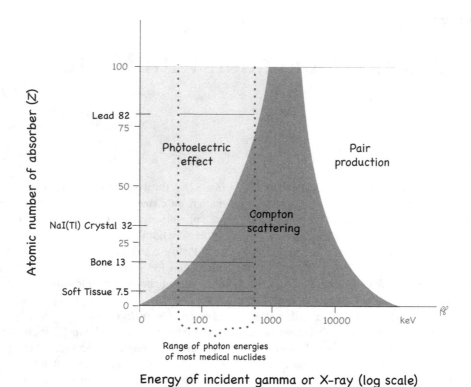

Figure 2.1 Predominant types of interaction for a range of incident photon energies and absorber atomic numbers.

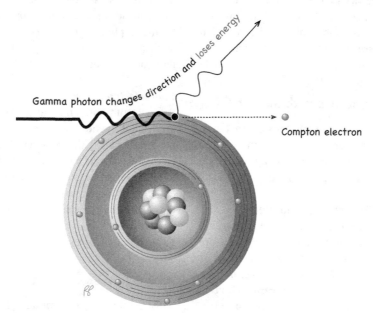

Figure 2.2 Compton scattering.

Attenuation of photons in matter

As a result of the interactions between photons and matter, the **intensity** of the **beam** (stream of photons), that is, the number of photons remaining in the beam, decreases as the beam passes through matter (Figure 2.5). This loss of photons is called **attenuation**; the matter through which the beam passes is referred to as the **attenuator**. Specifically, attenuation is the ratio of the intensity at the point where the beam exits the attenuator, I_{out}, to the intensity it had where it entered, I_{in}. The attenuation is an exponential function of the thickness x of the attenuator in centimeters. The fact that the function is exponential can be understood to mean that if half of the beam is lost in traversing the first centimeter of material, half of the remainder will be lost traversing the next centimeter, and so on. This resembles the exponential manner in which radioactivity decays with time. Expressed symbolically,

$$I_{out}/I_{in} = e^{-\mu x}$$

where μ, the **linear attenuation coefficient**, is a property of the attenuator. When, as is usually the case, thickness is given in centimeters, the linear attenuation coefficient is expressed as "per centimeter" or "cm^{-1}." As might be expected, the linear attenuation coefficient is greater for dense tissue such as bone than for soft tissue such as fat. In general, the linear attenuation coefficient depends on both the energy of the photons and on the average atomic number (Z) and the thickness of the attenuator. The lower the energy of the photons or the greater the average atomic number or thickness of the attenuator, the greater the attenuation (Figure 2.6).

A separate term, the **mass attenuation coefficient** (μ/ρ), is the linear attenuation coefficient divided by the density of the attenuator. When the density of a material is given in g/cm^3, the units of the mass attenuation coefficient are cm^2/g.

Absorption of radiation describes another aspect of the process of attenuation. Attenuation describes the weakening of the beam as it passes through matter. Absorption describes the transfer of energy from the beam to the matter.

Half-value and tenth-value layers

A material's effectiveness as a photon attenuator is described by the attenuation coefficient. An

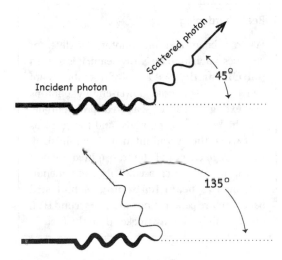

Figure 2.3 Angle of photon scattering.

Table 2.1 Predominant photon interactions in common materials at diagnostic energies

Material	Atomic number Z	Density (g/cm^3)	Predominant interaction
H$_2$O	7.4	1.0	Compton scattering
Soft tissue	7.5	1.0	Compton scattering
Glass (silica)	14	2.6	Compton scattering
O$_2$ (gas)	16	0.0014	Compton scattering
NaI (crystal)	32	3.7	Photoelectric effect
Lead	82	11.3	Photoelectric effect
Leaded glass	14, 82	4.8–6.2	Photoelectric effect

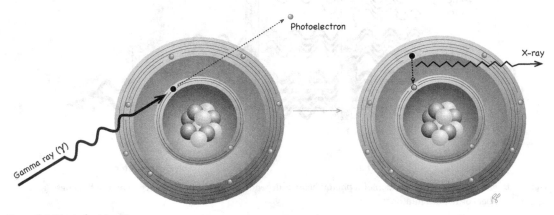

Figure 2.4 Photoelectric effect.

alternative descriptor, one that is more easily visualized, is the **half-value layer** (HVL), which is simply the thickness of a slab of the attenuator that will remove exactly one-half of the radiation of a beam. A second slab of the same thickness will remove half of the remainder (see the comment below regarding monoenergetic beams), leaving one-quarter of the original beam, and so forth. For a gamma photon of energy 100 keV, the HVL in soft tissue is about 4 cm [1].

For any attenuator, the HVL can be determined experimentally using a photon source and a suitable detector. For calculations involving attenuation of high-intensity radiation beams, an entirely

similar concept, the **tenth-value layer** (TVL), is useful. The TVL is the thickness of the attenuator that will transmit only one-tenth of the photons in the beam. For a monoenergetic beam (containing photons of identical energies) directed at a material, two such thicknesses will transmit only one-hundredth of the beam. If, however, the beam contains photons of different energies, this rule is not applicable (see the text box on beam hardening).

Table 2.2 lists the half- and tenth-value layers of lead for the photons emitted by some common medical radionuclides.

For a monoenergetic beam of photons, the linear attenuation coefficient μ is related to the HVL as follows:

$$\mu = 0.693/\text{HVL}$$

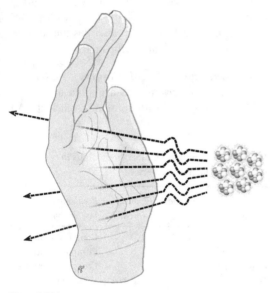

Figure 2.5 Attenuation.

Beam hardening

When a beam contains photons of different energies, such as in an X-ray beam, it is termed **polychromatic**. As a polychromatic beam penetrates a material, lower-energy photons are extinguished or scattered preferentially over higher-energy photons, and the result is that while the overall intensity is diminished, the average energy of the transmitted fraction of the beam is increased. This phenomenon is known as **beam hardening**. A hardened beam is more penetrating, and so a second HVL or TVL will be slightly thicker than the first.

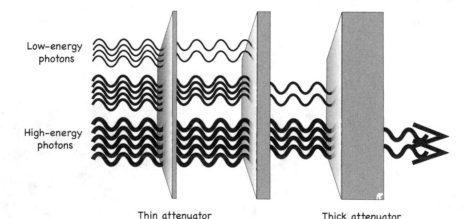

Low-energy photons

High-energy photons

Thin attenuator   Thick attenuator

Figure 2.6 The amount of attenuation of a photon beam is dependent on the photon energy and the thickness (and atomic number) of the attenuator.

Table 2.2 HVL and TVL of lead for photons from common medical nuclides

Nuclide	Gamma energy (keV)	Half-value layer (cm)	Tenth-value layer (cm)
^{99m}Tc	140	0.03	0.09
^{67}Ga	93, 185, 300, 393	0.02	0.27
^{123}I	159	0.04	0.12
^{131}I	364	0.22	0.74
^{18}F	511	0.39	1.3
^{111}In	172, 245	0.06	0.24

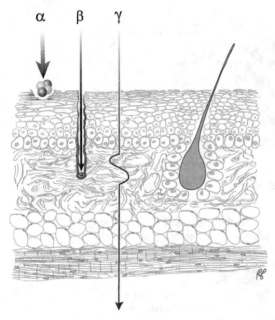

α   β   γ

Figure 2.7 Penetrating and nonpenetrating radiation.

The term **penetrating radiation** may be used to describe X-ray and gamma radiation, as these radiations have the potential to penetrate considerable thicknesses of a material. Although we have just described some of the many ways photons interact with matter, the likelihood of any of these interactions occurring over a short distance is small. An individual photon may travel several centimeters or farther into tissue before it interacts. In contrast, charged particles (i.e., alpha and beta particles) undergo many closely spaced interactions. This sharply limits their penetration through tissue as illustrated in a cross-section of epidermis in Figure 2.7.

Interaction of charged particles with matter

Because of the strong electrical force between a charged particle and the atoms of an absorber, charged particles can be stopped by matter with relative ease. Compared with photons, they transfer a greater amount of energy in a shorter distance and come to rest more rapidly. For this reason, they are referred to as **nonpenetrating radiation** (see the depiction of alpha and beta particles in Figure 2.7). In contrast to a photon of energy 100 keV, an electron of this energy would penetrate less than 0.00014 cm in soft tissue [1].

Excitation

Charged particles (alphas, betas, and positrons) interact with the electrons surrounding the atom's nucleus by transferring some of their kinetic energy to the electrons. The energy transferred from a low-energy particle is often only sufficient to bump an electron from an inner to an outer shell of the atom. This process is called excitation. Following excitation, the displaced electron promptly returns to the lower-energy shell, releasing its recently acquired energy as an X-ray in a process called de-excitation (Figure 2.8). Because the acquired energy is equal to the difference in the binding energies of the electron shells, and the binding energies of the electron shells are determined by the atomic structure of the element, the X-ray is referred to as a **characteristic X-ray**.

Ionization

Charged particles of sufficient energy may also transfer enough energy to an electron (generally one in an outer shell) to eject the electron from the atom. This process is called ionization (Figure 2.9). The hole in the outer shell is rapidly filled with an unbound electron. If an inner-shell electron is ionized (a much less frequent occurrence), an outer-shell electron will "drop" into the inner-shell hole and a characteristic X-ray will be emitted. Ionization is not limited to the interaction of charged particles and matter; the photoelectric effect and the Compton interaction are examples of photon interactions with matter that produce ionization.

Specific ionization

When radiation causes the ejection of an electron from an atom of an absorber, the resulting positively

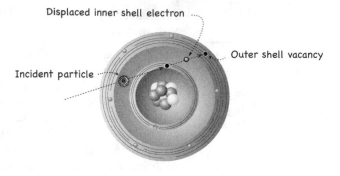

Excitation interaction

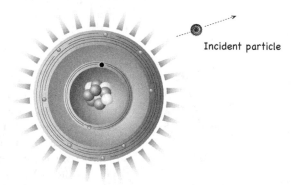

Excited (unstable) atom

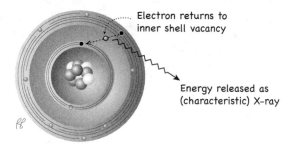

De-excitation

Figure 2.8 Excitation and de-excitation.

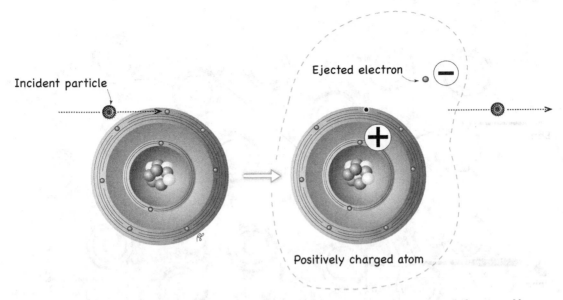

Figure 2.9 Ionization. The ejected electron and the positively charged atom are called an "ion pair" (demarcated by dashed line).

charged atom and free negatively charged electron are called an **ion pair** (Figure 2.9). The amount of energy transferred per ion pair created, W, is characteristic of the materials in the absorber. For example, approximately 33 eV (the range is 25–40 eV) is transferred to the absorber for each ion pair created in air or water. It is often convenient to refer to the number of ion pairs created per unit distance the radiation travels as its **specific ionization** (SI). Heavier particles with more charge (alpha particles) have a higher specific ionization than lighter particles with less charge (electrons).

Linear energy transfer

The **linear energy transfer** (LET) is the amount of energy transferred in a given distance by a particle moving through an absorber. Linear energy transfer is related to specific ionization:

$$LET = SI \times W$$

Alpha particles are classified as high-LET radiation, and beta particles and photons as low-LET radiation.

Range

The range is the distance radiation travels through an absorber. Particles that are lighter, have less charge (such as beta particles), and/or have greater energy travel farther than particles that are heavier,

have a greater charge (such as alpha particles), and/or have less energy (Figure 2.10).

In traversing an absorber, an electron loses energy at each interaction with the atoms of the absorber. The energy loss per interaction is variable. Therefore, the total distance traveled by electrons of the same energy can vary by as much as 3–4%. This variation in range is called the **straggling of the range**. The heavier alpha particles are not affected to a significant degree and demonstrate very little straggling of range.

Annihilation

This interaction in matter involves a positron (positive electron) and an electron (negatron). After a positron has transferred most of its kinetic energy by ionization and excitation, it combines with a free or loosely bound negative electron. Recall that electrons and positrons have equal mass but opposite electric charge. This interaction is explosive, as the combined mass of the two particles is instantly converted to energy in the form of two oppositely directed photons, each of energy 511 keV. This is referred to as an **annihilation reaction** (Figure 2.11). It is another example of the interchangeability of mass and energy described in Einstein's equation: energy equals mass times the speed of light squared, or $E = mc^2$ (Figure 2.12).

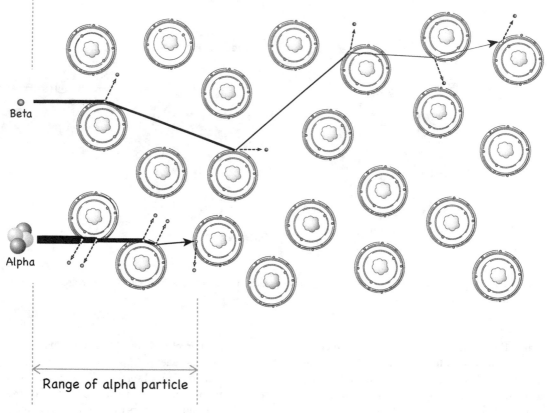

Figure 2.10 Particle range in an absorber.

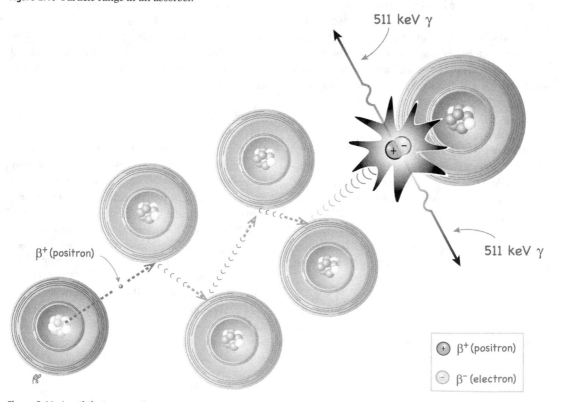

Figure 2.11 Annihilation reaction.

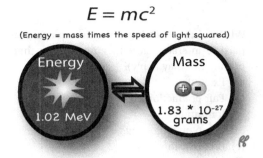

Figure 2.12 Einstein's theory of the equivalence of energy and mass.

Bremsstrahlung

Small charged particles such as electrons or positrons may be deflected by nuclei as they pass through matter, which may be attributed to the positive charge of the atomic nuclei. This type of interaction generates X-radiation known as **bremsstrahlung** (Figure 2.13), which in German means "braking radiation."

Reference

1. Shapiro J. *Radiation Protection. A Guide for Scientists, Regulators, and Physicians*, 4th edn. Cambridge, MA: Harvard University Press, 2002, pp. 42, 53.

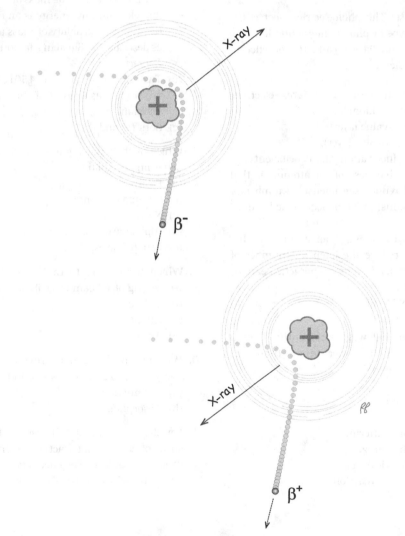

Figure 2.13 Bremsstrahlung. Beta particles (β^-) and positrons (β^+) that travel near the nucleus will be attracted or repelled by the positive charge of the nucleus, generating X-rays in the process.

Questions

1. Which of the following is true of the interaction of charged particles with matter?
   (a) Alpha particles have a higher LET than beta particles.
   (b) The range of alpha particles is generally greater than that of beta particles.
   (c) Alpha particles have a higher specific ionization than beta particles.

2. True or false: Bremsstrahlung is X-ray radiation emitted as a moving electron or positron slows down and is deflected in close proximity to a nucleus.

3. True or false: The photoelectric effect is the dominant type of photon interaction in tissue for the radionuclides used in the practice of nuclear medicine.

4. For each of the terms listed here, select the appropriate definition:
   (1) HVL (half-value layer).
   (2) TVL (tenth-value layer).
   (3) μ (mu) (linear attenuation coefficient).
       (a) The thickness of an attenuator that will reduce the intensity (number of photons) in a monoenergetic beam by 90%.
       (b) The thickness of an attenuator that will reduce the intensity (number of photons) in a monoenergetic beam by 50%.
       (c) 0.693/HVL.

5. Which of the following occur during photon interactions with matter (more than one answer may apply)?
   (a) Excitation.
   (b) Pair production.
   (c) Ionization.
   (d) Compton scattering.
   (e) Bremsstrahlung.
   (f) Photoelectric effect.
   (g) Annihilation reaction.

6. Which of the following occur during charged-particle interactions with atoms (more than one answer may apply)?
   (a) Excitation.
   (b) Pair production.
   (c) Ionization.
   (d) Compton scattering.
   (e) Bremsstrahlung.
   (f) Photoelectric effect.
   (g) Annihilation reaction.

7. Which of the following are true about the annihilation reaction?
   (a) The conversion of the mass of the positron and electron into energy is an example of the interchangeability of mass and energy as described by Einstein's famous equation $E = mc^2$.
   (b) Two oppositely directed 450 keV photons are emitted as a result of the annihilation reaction.
   (c) Both (a) and (b).

8. Which of the following are referred to as non-penetrating radiation?
   (a) Positrons.
   (b) Gamma photons.
   (c) X-rays.
   (d) Alpha particles.
   (e) Beta particles.

9. Which term refers to the loss of energy or weakening of a beam of radiation as it passes through matter?
   (a) Attenuation.
   (b) Absorption.

10. Which term is used to describe the transfer of energy from radiation to surrounding matter?
    (a) Attenuation.
    (b) Absorption.

11. You shield a sample of ^{99m}Tc using a 1 mm-thick sheet of lead. What fraction of emissions is blocked by the lead? The linear attenuation coefficient μ of lead for 140 keV photons is 23.1 cm^{-1}.

Answers

1. (a) and (c) are true, (b) is false; alpha particles have a shorter range than beta particles.
2. True.
3. False: Compton scattering is the dominant interaction.
4. (1) (b). (2) (a). (3) (c).
5. (b), (c), (d), (f).
6. (a), (c), (e), (g).
7. (a).
8. (a), (d), (e).
9. (a).
10. (b).
11. 0.21.

CHAPTER 3

Formation of Radionuclides

Many radionuclides exist in nature. An example is ^{14}C, which decays slowly with a half-life of 5700 years and is used to date fossils. The nuclides we use in nuclear medicine, however, are not naturally occurring but rather are made either by bombarding stable atoms or by splitting massive atoms. There are three basic types of equipment that are used to make medical nuclides: generators, cyclotrons, and nuclear reactors.

Generators

Generators are units that contain a radioactive **"parent" nuclide** with a relatively long half-life that decays to a short-lived **"daughter" nuclide**. The most commonly used generator is the technetium-99m (^{99m}Tc) generator (Figure 3.1), which consists of a heavily shielded column with molybdenum-99 (^{99}Mo, the parent) bound to the alumina of the column. The ^{99m}Tc (daughter) is "milked" (eluted) by drawing sterile saline through the column into a vacuum vial. The parent ^{99}Mo (small gray circles) remains on the column, but the daughter ^{99m}Tc (white circles) is washed away in the saline.

A generator like the one just described is frequently called a **cow**, the elution of the daughter nuclide is referred to as **milking**, and the surrounding lead is called a **pig**, a term used for any crude cast-metal container. Another generator that is used extensively for cardiac imaging is the $^{82}Sr-^{82}Rb$ generator. Its design and construction are very similar to those of the $^{99}Mo-^{99m}Tc$ generator but, owing to the 75s half-life of ^{82}Rb, the generator must be located on site—usually right next to a PET scanner, where the generator is eluted and the solution is infused into the patient in one automated step.

Table 3.1 describes the features of three common generators.

Activity curves for generators

The formal mathematical description of the time–activity behavior of parent and daughter radionuclides is complicated because it involves competition between the accumulation—caused by decay of the parent—and decay of the daughter. The curve describing the amount of daughter nuclide in a generator following elution has two segments. The first segment traces the period of rapid accumulation of the daughter nuclide and lasts for approximately four half-lives of the daughter nuclide (which, for ^{99m}Tc, is approximately 24 h). The second segment of the curve traces what is called the period of **equilibrium**, during which time the amount of daughter nuclide decreases as the parent nuclide decays.

Medical radionuclide generator systems, for practical reasons, have parent half-lives longer than the half-lives of their daughters—in most cases much longer. We classify generators into two groups: those in which the parent half-life is 10 to 100 times that of the daughter and those in which the parent half-life is more than 100 times that of the daughter. In the first group, the activity of the daughter during equilibrium decreases perceptibly over time (when time is measured in units of the daughter half-life). This is called **transient equilibrium**. On the other hand, the equilibrium segment of the

Essentials of Nuclear Medicine Physics and Instrumentation, Third Edition. Rachel A. Powsner, Matthew R. Palmer, and Edward R. Powsner.

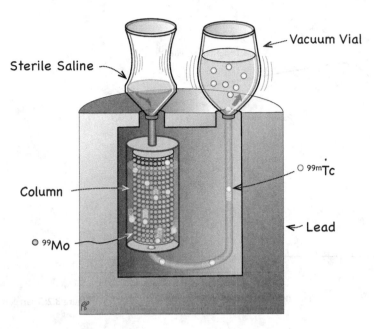

Sterile Saline

Vacuum Vial

Column

^{99m}Tc

^{99}Mo

Lead

Figure 3.1 Technetium-99m generator.

Table 3.1 Characteristics of three commonly used generators

Generator (parent–daughter)	Clinical uses of daughter nuclide	Half-life of parent ($T_{1/2\,p}$)	Half-life of daughter ($T_{1/2\,d}$)	$T_{1/2\,p}/T_{1/2\,d}$
^{99}Mo–^{99m}Tc (molybdenum-99–technetium-99m)	Used in most radiopharmaceuticals for nuclear studies	66 h	6 h	11
^{82}Sr–^{82}Rb (strontium-82–rubidium-82)	Cardiac perfusion imaging (PET)	25.5 days	75 s	29,000
^{68}Ge–^{68}Ga (germanium-82–gallium-82)	Neuroendocrine imaging (PET)	271 days	68 min	5,800

curve for the second group is relatively flat. This is called **secular equilibrium**.

Transient equilibrium

Transient equilibrium is illustrated in Figure 3.2. In this example, the half-life of the parent nuclide is approximately 10 times that of the daughter. Following an elution that removes all of the available daughter, the amount of the daughter nuclide increases rapidly until the activity of the daughter slightly exceeds that of the parent at about four to five half-lives. Thereafter the daughter activity declines at the same rate as the parent activity.

The preceding example of transient equilibrium is based on a decay scheme in which 100% of the parent nuclide decays to the daughter nuclide. However, in the commonly used ^{99}Mo–^{99m}Tc generator, only 86% of the parent molybendum-99 decays to the daughter technetium-99m; the remainder decays directly to technetium-99 (Figure 3.3). As a result, the activity of the ^{99m}Tc is always less than the activity of the ^{99}Mo (see Figure 3.3 again).

Secular equilibrium

For generators where the half-life of the parent is greater than 100 times that of the daughter

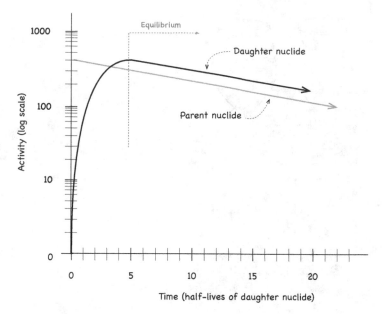

Figure 3.2 Transient equilibrium.

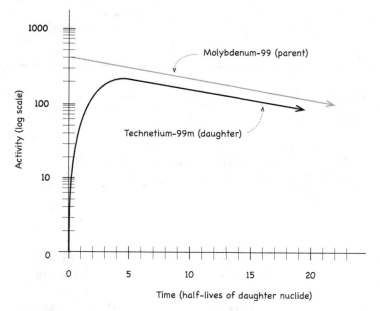

Figure 3.3 Transient equilibrium in a ^{99}Mo–^{99m}Tc generator.

nuclide, since we are interested in timescales on the order of the daughter half-life, we can just consider the parent nuclide to be stable. Secular equilibrium, like transient equilibrium, is achieved rapidly following an elution that removes all of the available daughter nuclide. Thereafter, the activity of the daughter nuclide is approximately equal to that of the parent. However, the decay curve of the parent appears to be flat, since the half-life of the parent is so much longer than that of the daughter nuclide. An example of secular equilibrium can be seen with the ^{82}Sr–^{82}Rb generator (see Figure 3.4).

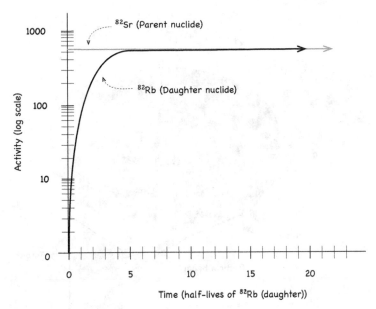

Figure 3.4 Secular equilibrium.

Cyclotrons

Cyclotrons are circular devices (Figure 3.5) in which charged particles such as protons and alpha particles are accelerated in a spiral path in a vacuum. A power supply provides a rapidly alternating voltage across the **dees** (the two halves of the circle). This produces a rapidly alternating electric field between the dees that accelerates the particles, which quickly acquire high kinetic energies. The particles spiral outward under the influence of the magnetic field until they have sufficient velocity, and are then deflected into a target.

A deflector is used to direct the particles out through a window in the cyclotron into a **target**. Some of the particles and some of the kinetic energy from these particles are incorporated into the nuclei of the atoms of the target. These energized (excited) nuclei are unstable.

Indium-111 (^{111}In) is produced in a cyclotron. The accelerated (bombarding) particles are protons. The target atoms are cadmium-112 (^{112}Cd). When a proton enters the nucleus of a ^{112}Cd atom, the ^{112}Cd is transformed into ^{111}In by discharging two neutrons. This reaction can be written as

Target atom (bombarding particle,

emitted particles) product nuclide

Cadmium-112 (proton, two neutrons) Indium-111

or

$$^{112}Cd(p,2n)^{111}In$$

Other examples of cyclotron reactions include $^{121}Sb(\alpha,2n)^{123}I$, $^{68}Zn(d,n)^{67}Ga$, and $^{10}B(d,n)^{11}C$, where the symbols α and d denote an alpha particles and a deuteron (proton plus neutron), respectively.

Reactors

Radionuclides for nuclear medicine are also produced in nuclear reactors. Some examples are ^{131}I, ^{133}Xe, and ^{99}Mo.

Reactor basics

A reactor is composed of **fuel rods** that contain large atoms (typically uranium-235, uranium-238, or plutonium-239) that are inherently unstable. These atoms undergo **fission** (see Figure 1.14). Two or three neutrons and approximately 200 MeV of heat energy are emitted during this process. These neutrons leave the nucleus with moderately high kinetic energies and are referred to as **fast neutrons**. The neutrons are slowed with a **moderator**

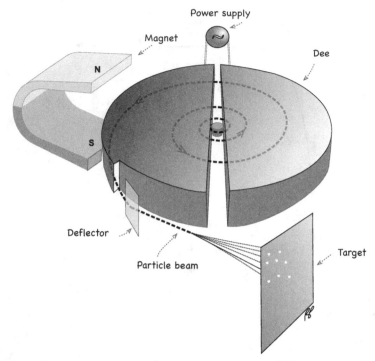

Figure 3.5 Cyclotron.

such as graphite, water, or heavy water. The resulting "very slow" neutrons, or **thermal neutrons**, and to a lesser extent the fast neutrons, in turn impact other fissionable atoms, causing their fission, and so forth (Figure 3.6). If this **chain reaction** were to grow unchecked, the mass would explode. To maintain control, cadmium **control rods** are inserted to absorb the neutrons in the reactor. They can be inserted further or withdrawn to control the speed of the reaction.

Medical nuclides are made in reactors by the processes of fission and neutron capture.

Kinetic energy

"Kinetic" means "motion." The form of energy attributable to the motion of an object is its kinetic energy. Kinetic energy is related to both the mass (m) and velocity (v) of the object; specifically, it is equal to $(1/2)mv^2$. A moving car has kinetic energy; a parked car does not. A speeding car contains a great deal of kinetic energy that can be dissipated rapidly as heat, noise, and the destruction of metal in a collision.

Fission

In this process, the desired radionuclide is one of the **fission fragments** of a heavy element $(Z > 92)$, either an atom of the fuel itself or an atom of a target placed inside the reactor. This **by-product** is chemically separated from the other fission fragments. The fission reaction is denoted as

$$^{235}\text{Uranium (neutron, fission) daughter}$$
$$\text{nuclide}$$

For example, the formation of iodine-131 and that of molybdenum-99 are written as

$$^{235}\text{U}(n,f)^{131}\text{I and }^{235}\text{U}(n,f)^{99}\text{Mo}$$

Neutron capture

In neutron capture, the target atom captures a neutron. The new atom is radioactive and emits gamma photons or charged particles to produce a daughter nuclide (Figure 3.7). A gamma photon is emitted following capture of a thermal neutron. This reaction is written as

$$\text{Target (neutron, gamma) daughter nuclide}$$

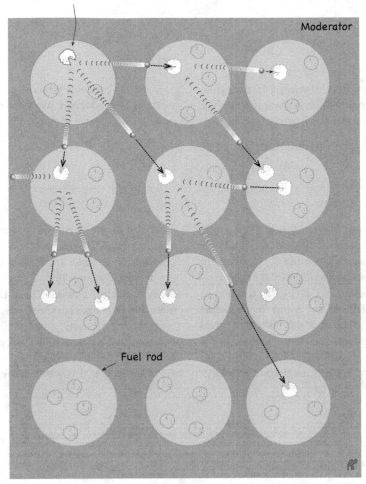

Figure 3.6 Chain reaction involving ²³⁵U and slow neutrons.

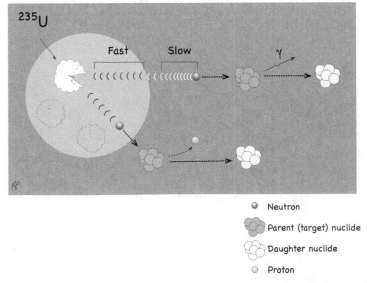

Figure 3.7 Neutron capture. Capture of thermal (slow) neutron with gamma emission (top); fast-neutron capture with proton emission (bottom).

For example,

$$^{98}\text{Mo}(n,\gamma)^{99}\text{Mo}$$

When the target atom captures a fast neutron, a proton can be emitted. This capture reaction is a type of **transmutation** and is symbolized as

Target (neutron, proton) daughter nuclide

For example,

$$^{32}\text{S}(n,p)^{32}\text{P}$$

A list of common medical nuclides and their methods of production, modes of decay, and decay products is provided in Appendix A.

Radionuclide production

There is often more than one way to make a radionuclide. For example, ^{111}In is most commonly made in a cyclotron using the $^{112}\text{Cd}(p,2n)^{111}\text{In}$ reaction, but it can also be made from a cadmium-111 target using the $^{111}\text{Cd}(p,n)^{111}\text{In}$ reaction or from a silver-109 target using the reaction $^{109}\text{Ag}(\alpha,2n)^{111}\text{In}$. The trade-offs involve the relative efficiencies of production for various cyclotron energies and the issues involved in separating and purifying the product. In general, bombardment of a target by charged particles in a cyclotron increases the charge-to-mass ratio, and so nuclei in the product are likely to be charge-rich (neutron-poor) and thus decay via beta-plus decay or electron capture. This is the reason that most PET radionuclides are produced using a cyclotron. Conversely, bombarding a target with neutrons in a reactor tends to increase the mass of the target nuclei, rendering them neutron-rich and thus likely to decay by beta-minus decay.

Questions

1. Which of the following statements are true about medical radionuclide generators?
   (a) The parent nuclide always has a shorter half-life than the daughter nuclide.
   (b) If the $T_{1/2}$ of the parent nuclide is 50 times greater than the $T_{1/2}$ of the daughter nuclide, the equilibrium portion of the activity curve is basically flat and is categorized as "secular" equilibrium.
   (c) The parent nuclide is less tightly bound to the column than the daughter nuclide is.
   (d) All of the above.
   (e) None of the above.

2. True or false: During an equilibrium state within a ^{99}Mo–^{99m}Tc generator, the total activity of ^{99m}Tc is always less than the total activity of ^{99}Mo because 14% of ^{99}Mo decays directly to ^{99}Tc, bypassing the metastable state.

3. Which of the following is an example of a generator that reaches secular equilibrium?
   (a) ^{99}Mo–^{99m}Tc.
   (b) ^{82}Sr–^{82}Rb.

4. Associate each of the following terms (a) through (k) with the most appropriate of the three methods of nuclide production listed here:
   (1) Generator.
   (2) Cyclotron.
   (3) Reactor.
       (a) Moderator.
       (b) Chain reaction.
       (c) Thermal neutron.
       (d) Dee.
       (e) Control rod.
       (f) Target.
       (g) Cow.
       (h) Pig.
       (i) Column.
       (j) Elution.
       (k) By-product.

5. Associate each of the following nuclear reactions (a) through (d) with the most appropriate of the three production methods listed:
   (1) Cyclotron.
   (2) Fission reaction (reactor).
   (3) Neutron capture (reactor).
   (a) ^{111}Cd(p,n)^{111}In.
   (b) ^{68}Zn(d,n)^{67}Ga.
   (c) ^{235}U(n,f)^{99}Mo.
   (d) ^{98}Mo(n,γ)^{99}Mo

6. F-18 is produced:
   (a) In a generator.
   (b) In a cyclotron.
   (c) From by-product material of nuclear fission.
   (d) By neutron bombardment in a nuclear reactor.

7. Mo-99 is produced:
   (a) In a generator.
   (b) In a cyclotron.
   (c) From by-product material of nuclear fission.
   (d) By neutron bombardment in a nuclear reactor.

8. Tc-99m is produced:
   (a) In a generator.
   (b) In a cyclotron.
   (c) From by-product material of nuclear fission.
   (d) By neutron bombardment in a nuclear reactor.

9. The half-life of ^{99m}Tc is 6 h and the half-life of ^{99}Mo is 66 h. At 8 AM Monday morning, a Tc/Mo generator is eluted and the yield is 100 mCi ^{99m}Tc. Approximately how much ^{99m}Tc will we be able to elute from the generator on Friday at 8 AM?
   (a) Essentially zero, since more than 10 half-lives have elapsed.
   (b) 36 mCi.
   (c) 100 mCi.
   (d) 50 mCi.

Answers

1. (e) None of the above: (a) the parent half-life is always longer than the daughter half-life; (b) if the half-life of the parent is between 10 and 100 times greater than the half-life of the daughter, the activity curve is downward-sloping and the equilibrium is termed "transient"; and (c) the daughter nuclide is less tightly bound, and therefore it can be removed or eluted for use.
2. True.

3. (b).
4. (a), (b), (c), (e), (f), and (k) are terms for reactors; (d) and (f) are terms for cyclotrons; (g), (h), (i), and (j) are terms for generators.
5. (a) (1). (b) (1). (c) (2). (d) (3).
6. (b) In a cyclotron.
7. (d) By neutron bombardment in a nuclear reactor.
8. (a) In a generator.
9. (b) 36 mCi.

CHAPTER 4

Nonscintillation Detectors

Because we generally cannot sense the presence of radioactivity, electronic equipment has been developed to detect ionizing radiation (both particles and photons). This chapter explores the common types of nonscintillation radiation detectors used in a nuclear medicine department; the next chapter discusses scintillation detectors.

Gas-filled detectors

Theory of operation

Gas-filled detectors function by measuring the ionization that radiation produces within the gas. There are several types of detectors that operate on this general principle, but they differ greatly in their details of construction and in the manner in which the radiation-produced ionization is gauged. As might be expected, each type has one or more applications for which it is best suited.

One important factor determining the applicability of gas-filled detectors is the nature and state of the gas itself. For example, because the molecules of any gas are relatively widely separated, they are more likely to be ionized by strongly ionizing charged particles, such as alpha and beta radiation, than by gamma (photon) radiation. Partially for this reason, gas-filled detectors are usually used to monitor alpha and beta radiation, although with appropriate design a gas-filled detector can also be used to measure photon (gamma or X-ray) radiation.

Principles of measurement

Charge neutralization

Perhaps one of the simplest and oldest methods for quantifying the ionization produced in a gas detector is visual observation of the filament of an electroscope. An example is provided by the pocket dosimeter, illustrated later in this chapter, which contains a small gas-filled chamber within which a thin filament of wire is attached to a metal frame. When positively charged, the filament is repelled by the frame, which also carries a positive charge. The filament is observed to return to its resting position as the charge is neutralized by the radiation-produced ions. The greater the amount of incoming radiation, the closer the filament moves toward the neutral position.

Charge flow

Measuring current: A related approach is to measure the flow of the charges that ionizing radiation produces in a gas-filled detector. The ions produced by the radiation are charged particles. The negative particle is either a free electron or an oxygen or nitrogen molecule that has absorbed a free electron. The positive particle is a molecule of gas that has lost an electron.

The gas-filled detector has both a positive and a negative electrode (Figure 4.1). As shown in a cross section in Figure 4.2, the potential difference

Essentials of Nuclear Medicine Physics and Instrumentation, Third Edition. Rachel A. Powsner, Matthew R. Palmer, and Edward R. Powsner.

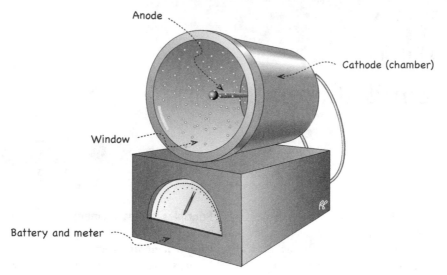

Anode

Cathode (chamber)

Window

Battery and meter

Figure 4.1 Simple gas-filled detector.

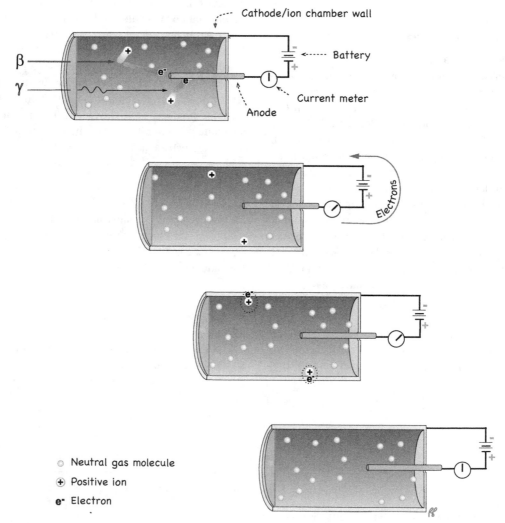

Cathode/ion chamber wall

β

γ

Battery

e⁻

e

Current meter

Anode

Electrons

⊙ Neutral gas molecule

⊕ Positive ion

e⁻ Electron

Figure 4.2 Gas-filled detector. The presence of ionizing radiation is detected by a deflection of the current meter.

between them is maintained by a battery. The positive and negative ions produced in the gas by the radiation move in opposite directions, positive ions toward the cathode and negative ions toward the anode. This movement of ions (charges) is an electric current, which can be detected by a sensitive meter. The current between the electrodes is a measure of the amount of incoming radiation. The **ionization chamber**, about which more is said later in this chapter, is a practical instrument that functions in this way.

Counting pulses of current: The alternative to measuring the current is counting the individual pulses produced as each individual charged particle or photon enters the gas. The **Geiger counter** is an example of this type of detector. The rate at which counts occur in such detectors is a direct measure of the amount of incoming radiation.

The process of ionization, collection of the charges produced, and recording of the count takes place very quickly, but it is far from instantaneous. Time is required for the ions to reach their respective electrodes and for the detector to return to its resting state. What transpires in this time depends on the construction of the detector, the kind of gases it contains, and the strength of the applied voltage. Although all three factors determine the characteristics of the detector, it is instructive to examine the role of the applied voltage in more detail.

Characteristics of the major regions of applied voltage across a gas-filled detector

Low

In a gas-filled detector, the magnitude of the voltage between the electrodes determines the type of the response to each charged particle or photon. When the voltage between the electrodes is relatively low, the field within the gas is weak and many of the ions simply recombine, leaving only a small fraction to reach the electrodes. Little if any charge flows between the electrodes, and the meter in the external circuit remains at zero.

At somewhat higher voltages, referred to as the **ionization region** (Figure 4.3), most of the ions that are formed reach the electrodes. A further small increase in the voltage does not increase the current once the voltage is sufficient to collect 100% of the ions formed. The brief pulse of current generated by ionizing radiation entering the chamber ceases until the next charged particle or photon enters the gas. This current is small, and difficult to count as an individual event.

In this region, the current is relatively independent of small increases in voltage. It is, however, affected by the type of radiation. An alpha particle, because it carries two units of charge and is relatively massive, produces many ion pairs while traveling a short distance in the gas; a beta particle, which is much lighter and carries only a single charge, produces fewer ion pairs per unit distance traveled; and a photon, because it carries neither charge nor mass, creates even fewer ion pairs. In any case, practically all of the ion pairs that are created are collected on the electrodes because the applied voltage creates a strong enough electric field to prevent recombination.

In small detectors, some of the ionization from beta radiation and much or even most of the ionization from photon radiation may escape detection. In this situation, the current following irradiation by an alpha particle will be much larger than that caused by a beta particle of similar energy, and the currents following both of these particles will be larger than that caused by photon radiation of similar energy.

Intermediate

With further increase in voltage, the detector passes into the next region of operation (see Figure 4.3). In this so-called **proportional region**, a new phenomenon is observed—**gas amplification** (Figure 4.4). Accelerated more intensely toward the positive electrode at this higher voltage, the electrons produced by the radiation (called primary particles) travel so rapidly that they themselves are able to ionize some of the previously neutral gas molecules. This process, similar to that produced by the original radiation particle, can be imagined as a speeding electron knocking out a molecular electron (a new negative ion) and leaving behind a positively charged gas molecule (a new positive ion). The newly separated electrons (called **delta** or secondary particles) also accelerate toward the positive electrode and, in turn, ionize additional gas molecules. The pulse of charge started by the incoming radiation is greatly amplified by this brief chain reaction.

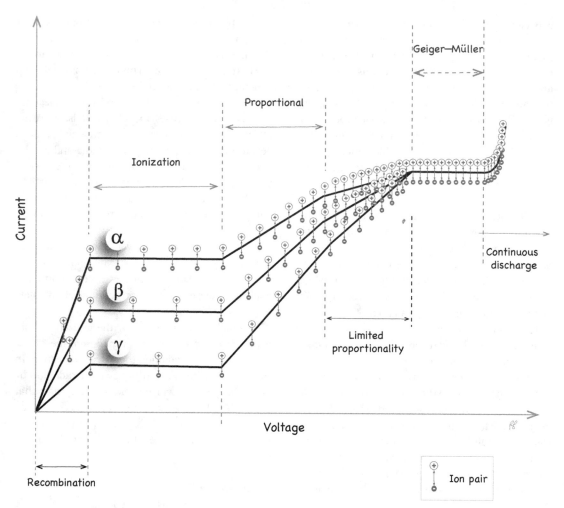

Figure 4.3 Current as a function of applied voltage in a gas detector. The regions of interest include the ionization, proportional, and Geiger–Müller regions.

In this region, the current produced is proportional to the number of ion pairs produced by the incoming radiation. The current is higher for an alpha particle than for a beta, and the currents for both are higher than for a photon. Because of gas amplification, the total number of ion pairs, primary plus secondary, is much higher than in the low-voltage ionization region. This resulting pulse of current is large enough to detect as an individual, countable event.

High

For detectors operating at still higher voltages, above the proportional region, the pulse of current

is larger but becomes independent of the number of ions produced by the initial event. As the voltage is increased, a point is reached at which most of the gas within the detector is massively involved in multiple, successive ionizations (Figure 4.5). Once all the gas is involved, no greater gas amplification is possible, so that any further increases in voltage have little effect on the size of the pulse of current. This is the so-called **Geiger** (or **Geiger–Müller**) region. A detector operating in this region is called a Geiger counter, or Geiger–Müller counter, after its early developers. In the Geiger region, not only is the size of the current pulse almost independent of small changes in voltage, but the size of the pulse is

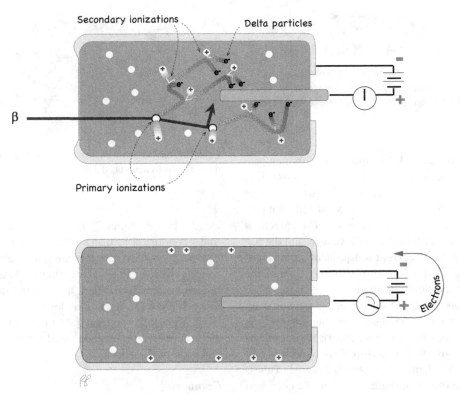

Figure 4.4 Proportional counter. The voltage causes gas amplification by giving electrons separated during primary ionization enough energy to cause secondary ionization.

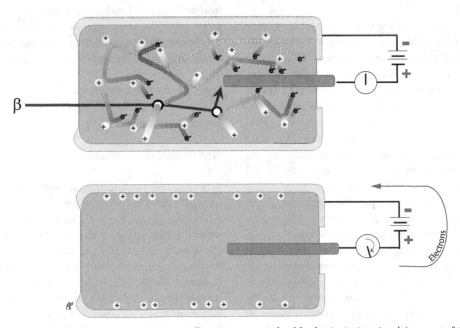

Figure 4.5 Geiger counter. The primary radiation rapidly triggers a cascade of further ionizations involving most of the gas.

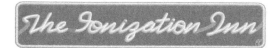

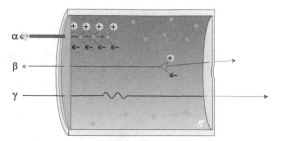

Figure 4.6 Continuous discharge. The voltage applied to a neon sign is high enough to generate spontaneous ionization that continues until the power is turned off.

Figure 4.7 Ionization by alpha particles, beta particles, and photons in a gas-filled detector.

also independent of the amount of ionization produced by the incoming radiation. In other words, in the Geiger region the current produced by a charged particle or photon is large compared with that produced in the proportional region. The current is independent of fluctuations in voltage, and the size of each pulse of current is dependent on the characteristics of the detector itself rather than of the incoming particle or photon.

Voltages above the Geiger region are not used, because even in the absence of the radiation the counter is designed to detect, there is a spontaneous and **continuous ionization** of gas molecules that stops only when the voltage is lowered. This is similar to the visible ionization seen in a neon sign (Figure 4.6). With such high voltages, the device is not useful as a radiation detector.

Sensitivity

Intrinsic

A gas-filled detector will respond to virtually every radiation event that causes ionization in the gas. To be detected, a particle or photon must be energetic enough to cross the detector face into the sensitive volume of gas, but must not be so energetic that it will pass right through the gas without causing any ionization. The first limitation is important for low-energy alpha or beta particles, which have only limited ability to penetrate the "window" of the detector, but once inside ionize strongly. The second is a consideration for high-energy photons, which penetrate easily but may pass through the detector, causing little or no ionization (Figure 4.7). Sensitivity for charged particles (alpha or beta) can be increased by using thin, penetrable materials for the detector window such as a thin sheet of mica or, for greatest sensitivity, by actually placing the radioactive sample inside the sensitive volume. Sensitivity for moderately high-energy photons is improved by increasing the size of the sensitive volume or, equiv-

alently, by "cramming" in more gas molecules under pressure or by using a thicker window.

Typical gas-filled detectors are sensitive to alpha particles with energies greater than 3–4 MeV, beta radiation above 50–100 keV, and gamma radiation above 5–7 keV. The upper limit for gamma or X-ray radiation depends on the type and pressure of the gas and the type of material used for the window and walls of the detector.

Geometric

The larger the window and the closer the source, the more radiation will enter the detector. At long distances from compact sources, the amount of radiation reaching the detector decreases with the square of the distance. The controlling factor, aside from absorption of radiation in the intervening air, is the portion of the source seen by the window. As can be seen in Figure 4.8, this is the fraction of the sphere subtended (or seen) by the window.

Types of gas-filled detectors

Ionization chambers

Structure and characteristics

Structure: The ionization chamber, in its simplest form, is a gas-filled can (the gas is usually air) with a radiation-permeable end (the window), a central wire, a meter, and a battery (see Figure 4.1). The gas is most often at normal atmospheric pressure, but the chamber may be filled under pressure, as discussed under Geiger counters below. A thin window at one end of the can admits radiation. A battery or power supply maintains the central wire at a positive potential relative to the surrounding

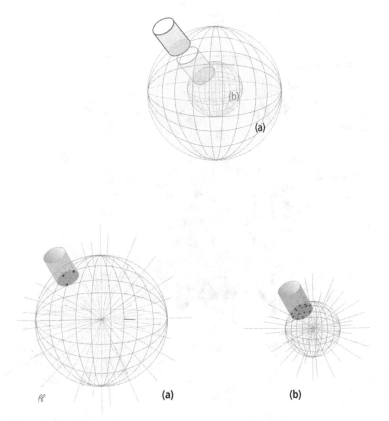

Figure 4.8 Geometric efficiency of detectors. The closer the detector is to the source (b), the greater the number of photons that will cross the detector window.

walls of the can, which act as the negative electrode. The magnitude of the voltage is set relatively low to ensure operation in the ionization region, hence the name "ionization chamber" (see Figure 4.3). A sensitive meter to measure the current of ions completes the device.

Function: The ionization chamber is not ordinarily used to count discrete radiation events but rather to measure the average number of ionizations per minute occurring within the gas. If the events are sufficiently infrequent, the attached meter may be observed to move up a short distance as a particle or photon of radiation triggers the detector, and to fall back slowly in the interval before the next event.

Sensitivity: The lower limit of sensitivity for an ionization chamber is determined by the sensitivity of the meter used to measure the current. In terms of radiation exposure, sensitivity down to less

than 1 mR/hr for low- and moderate-energy photons (10 keV to 1 MeV) is available with standard survey meters and dosimeters.

Energy independence: In the ionization region of operation, the electrodes collect practically all of the ion pairs formed in the gas. Because the number of ionizations is almost directly proportional to the energy of the incoming radiation, the current that results is a measure of the rate at which energy is being deposited within the gas by the ionizing radiation. The rate of ionization, the consequent current, and the radiation dose are all similarly dependent on the energy of the incoming particles or photons. As a result, at least for an ideal ionization chamber, the meter reading gives a reliable measure of the radiation dose rate. Note, however, that this reliability has its limits. As alluded to above, at very low energies the radiation may not even penetrate the ion chamber, and at very high energies the radiation

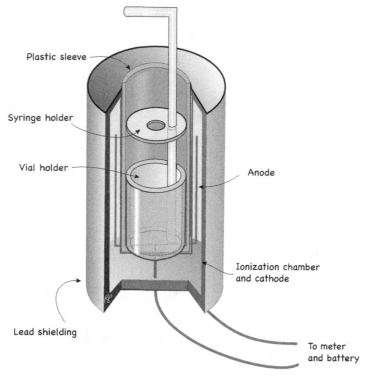

Plastic sleeve

Syringe holder

Vial holder

Anode

Ionization chamber
and cathode

Lead shielding

To meter
and battery

Figure 4.9 Dose calibrator.

may pass completely through the device without having many ionizing interactions with the gas.

Applications

Dose calibrator: A dose calibrator is most frequently used in the nuclear medicine department as a table-top ionization chamber to confirm that the correct amount of activity has been dispensed before a dose of radiopharmaceutical is administered (Figure 4.9). The dose calibrator consists of an ionization chamber surrounding an open well. The walls of the well are permeable to photons. The current produced in the circuitry is proportional to the number of primary ionizations in the chamber. The amount of current is registered as radioactivity in megabecquerels or millicuries. The dose calibrator can report only the activity, not the type of radiation or radiopharmaceutical.

The accuracy of the reading is affected by such factors as the type of dose container, its proper placement in the dose calibrator, and the calibration and regular recalibration of the instrument itself. Because of the importance of administering the correct amount of activity to patients, there are strictly enforced rules for the use and calibration of dose calibrators. These are discussed in Chapter 9.

Survey meter: When an ionization chamber is used as a survey meter, the current reading is usually interpreted as the average intensity of radiation in roentgens (R) per hour. For example, a survey meter might register a 30 mR/h exposure rate at one meter from a person who was treated with 370 MBq (10 mCi) of ^{131}I. The roentgen is defined in terms of ionization produced in air, and it is no coincidence that the ionization chamber can be used for the measurement of radiation intensity in roentgens.

The roentgen (R)

The roentgen is a measurement of gamma or X-ray radiation exposure in air, not tissue. One roentgen is the quantity of radiation that will produce 2.58×10^{-4} coulombs (C) of charge (or 2×10^9 ion pairs) per kilogram of dry air under standard conditions.

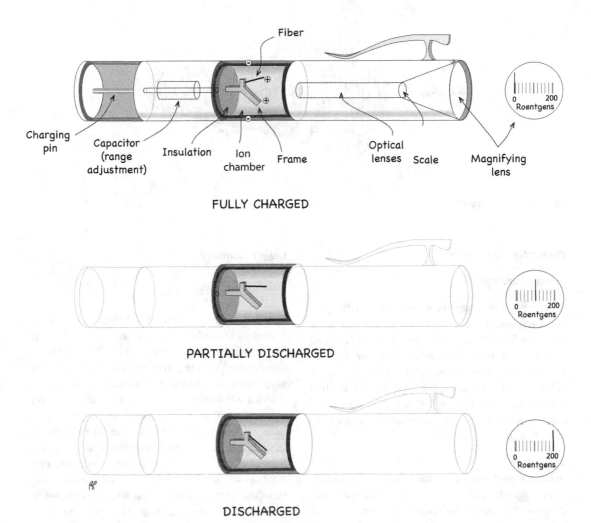

Figure 4.10 Pocket dosimeter. Ions produced in the gas neutralize the charge on the filament and frame and the filament returns toward its neutral position. Adapted from a drawing of the FEMA dosimeter, courtesy of Federal Emergency Management Agency, Washington, DC, USA.

Pocket dosimeters: A small ionization chamber is the heart of the classic pocket dosimeter. For this application, a small, straight filament, insulated from the walls of the chamber, is mounted within the ionization chamber (Figure 4.10). To prepare the chamber for use, a positive charge is placed on the filament by a charger that briefly connects the positive terminal of a battery to the filament. When charged, the positive filament is repelled by the positively charged frame. When radiation penetrates the walls of the chamber, the gas is ionized and the ions are attracted to the frame and fiber or to the walls of the chamber, and this partially neutralizes their charge. The filament is less strongly repelled by the frame and begins to move toward a neutral position. The position of the filament can be viewed through a lens against a scale on the end of the chamber, calibrated in roentgens or rads. Properly insulated from the case of the chamber, the positive charge can remain on the filament for hours.

Pocket dosimeters of this type are relatively inexpensive and can be used to measure exposures to photons in the range of zero to several hundred millirads. A separate charging device is required.

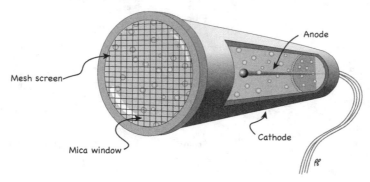

Figure 4.11 Geiger probe.

Proportional counters

Structure and characteristics

Chamber and filling gas: In its construction, the proportional counter is very similar to the ionization chamber. The filling gas is more likely to be argon or an argon–methane mixture than air, but the essential difference between them is the higher voltage and the resulting gas amplification. For this reason, the incoming radiation causes a pulse of current large enough to be registered as an individual count.

Applications as survey meter: The proportional counter is particularly suitable when it is important to distinguish between various types of radiation. Because the size of the pulse from a proportional counter is proportional to the initial ionization, alpha particles, which ionize more heavily than beta particles, produce larger pulses, and this difference can be used to distinguish between them.

Counting low-energy particles may require very close proximity of the detector to the sample. Proportional counters can be built for this type of counting with no window or only a very thin, somewhat leaky membrane between the sample and the gas of the chamber. In the windowless type, the sample is placed directly within the gas-filled chamber. A continuous flow of gas through the detector compensates for any loss of gas as samples are inserted or, in the case of the type with a thin window, for any gas that leaks through the membrane. Gas-flow counting is relatively exacting and, for many purposes, has been replaced by the less exacting liquid scintillation counting method.

Geiger counters

Structure and characteristics

The tube and the filling gas: The Geiger counter is an ionization chamber that operates at a relatively high applied voltage (Figure 4.11). The chamber is usually filled with argon containing traces of other gases such as a halogen or methane, although a detector will function with a filling as simple as dry air. The sensitive end of the probe is generally a mica window protected by an external metal mesh. In some applications, the thin window of the ionization chamber is covered by an aluminum cap. Photons striking the cap knock out secondary electrons that in turn ionize the gas within the chamber. The walls of the chamber may also function similarly.

The gas in the chamber may be filled to atmospheric pressure or may be pressurized to increase sensitivity. At higher pressures, usually a few times normal atmospheric pressure, the number of gas molecules "crammed" into the chamber is greater. This raises the probability that incoming radiation will encounter and ionize a gas molecule within the chamber. Pressurization is particularly useful for photon radiation for which the energy is high enough, and therefore the range of the photons in the gas long enough, to allow a photon to pass completely through an unpressurized chamber without encountering and ionizing a gas molecule. The Geiger counter cannot distinguish between types of radiation, because each interaction of the radiation with the gas causes maximum ionization.

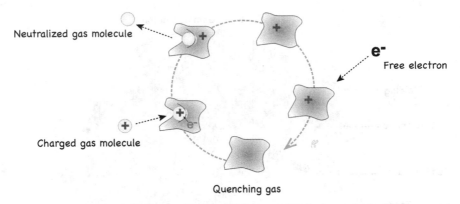

Neutralized gas molecule

e⁻
Free electron

Charged gas molecule

Quenching gas

Figure 4.12 Quenching materials within the gas chamber rapidly neutralize the positively charged gas particles.

Quenching: The gas multiplication that characterizes the Geiger region causes a single incoming radiation event to give a large current pulse, but gas amplification carries the disadvantage that the discharge, once started by the radiation, is likely to sustain itself indefinitely. While the discharge continues, the detector is not affected by any further incoming radiation; it is effectively paralyzed (this **dead time** lasts 100–$500\,\mu s$ for Geiger counters). The discharge must be quenched before the tube can count again. The two common methods of **quenching** are to quickly drop the applied voltage or to add a quenching material to the filling gas. The latter serves to quench the discharge by absorbing the kinetic energy of the electrons and facilitating their recombination with the positive ions (Figure 4.12). Halogen compounds and small organic molecules such as methane are commonly used for this purpose. Whatever method is used, quenching is transparent to the user.

Applications: The Geiger counter has long been the most widely used of the gas-filled detectors. Its principal uses are the monitoring of areas such as nuclear medicine laboratories for radiation and the detection of contamination. When used as a **radiation monitor** to detect individual photons or measure their rate (usually referred to as counts and count rate, respectively), the Geiger counter is relatively independent of the energy of the photons. This is true provided that the photons are sufficiently energetic to enter the counting chamber

but not so energetic that they pass through it without interacting. When a Geiger counter is used as a **survey meter** to measure the exposure rate, usually in milliroentgens per hour, the meter reading is strongly affected by the energy of the photons. For low-energy photons, typically those below $100\,keV$, the actual exposure rate is only a fraction of the reading displayed on the meter. The reason for this is that the counter detects individual photons, not their energy, whereas the exposure rate depends on both the energy and flux of photons. The usual meter is calibrated for photons of moderate or even high energy such as those from ^{137}Cs or ^{60}Co. It must be recalibrated if the energy of the photons is expected to be very different from that used for the factory calibration.

Sensitivity: The Geiger counter can be expected to respond to any individual particle or photon whose energy is high enough to permit it to penetrate into the chamber but low enough that it does not, or is unlikely to, pass through without ionizing any gas molecules. From this, it is apparent that geometric considerations—the size and shape of the detector and its distance from the source—can be the most important factors limiting sensitivity.

For monitoring radiation of low intensity, the sensitivity is further limited by the background count. The count rate of the monitored radiation must be sufficient to increase the total significantly above the background. For radiation of high intensity, the sensitivity may be limited by the dead time

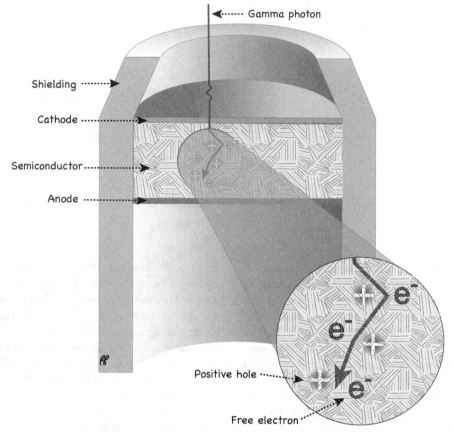

Figure 4.13 Semiconductor detector. Photons entering the detector create electron-hole pairs.

of the counter, which, as described above, is the time before one discharge has been quenched and the tube is able to count another event.

Semiconductor detectors

Semiconductors are crystalline materials with fewer mobile electrons than in a metallic material. As a result, the flow of electrical charge in these materials is more restricted than that in a metal such as copper, hence the name "semiconductors." **Semiconductor detectors** can be thought of as functionally equivalent to gas detectors but with all the advantages of a solid material. Similarly to what happens when radiation interacts with electrons of gas molecules, the atomic electrons in these solids can be "dislodged" by ionizing radiation. Instead of positively charged gas molecules, positive "holes"

are created in the crystalline structure (Figure 4.13). The electrons and holes migrate within the semiconductor as they are attracted to the anode and cathode attached to opposite sides of the detector (Figure 4.14).

The primary advantage of using solid materials instead of gases for detectors is their much higher density. The higher the density of a material, the more likely the interaction of incoming radiation with atoms of the material. In addition, the electrons in a semiconductor are less tightly bound to their atoms than the electrons in the atoms of gas molecules. It takes only 2–3 eV to "release" an electron in a semiconductor material, compared with approximately 35 eV to release an electron in air. This means that for any incoming radiation, there is a much greater yield of charges (positive holes and negative electrons) in a semiconductor than in

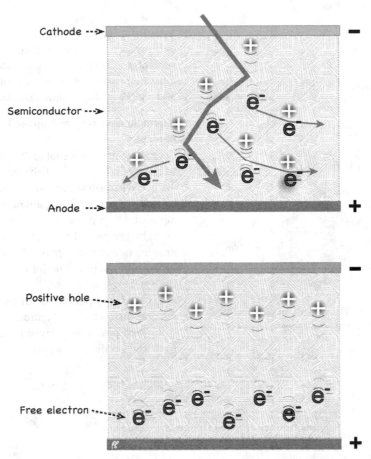

Figure 4.14 Electrons and positive holes formed by primary and secondary ionizations migrate in the field created by the anode and cathode.

air (or any other gas) of a similar volume. As a consequence, a smaller volume of solid material is needed, which allows the production of much smaller detectors.

A few of the many semiconductor compounds that are available for use are cadmium telluride (CdTe), cadmium zinc telluride (CdZnTe), and zinc telluride (ZnTe). Because of the high cost of manufacturing semiconductor materials, they have been used mainly in specialty applications such as intraoperative probes, although recently they have begun to appear in imaging systems.

Photographic and luminescent detectors

There are several types of radiosensitive materials that are typically used to measure the cumulative exposure received by personnel working with radioactivity. These materials are encased in plastic and worn by the user in either badge or ring form. Unlike the pen dosimeter, which can be read by the user, these badges must be sent to an outside laboratory for interpretation.

Photographic detectors

The **film badge** depicted in Figure 4.15 is one such detector. It is simply a plastic holder containing film that is radiosensitive. Strips of materials of different densities (such as aluminum, cadmium, and lead) are placed within the badge in the space in front of the film. These strips attenuate the incoming radiation and reduce the degree of exposure of the film located immediately behind the strip. As discussed in Chapter 2, the amount of attenuation is dependent

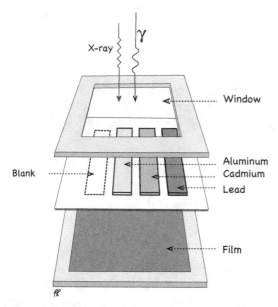

Figure 4.15 Film badge. The strips of metal absorbers assist in estimating the type and energy of radiation exposure.

on the type of radiation (alpha, beta, gamma, or X-ray), the energy of the radiation, and the density of the absorber. By comparing the amounts of exposure of the film behind each strip (including a fourth uncovered area), some estimate of the type and energy of the radiation can be made.

Thermoluminescent and optically luminescent detectors

Crystalline materials that emit light when exposed to energy (in the form of light, heat, radiation, etc.) are called **luminescent**. Luminescent crystals that can absorb energy from gamma rays, X-rays, and alpha and beta particles and then emit the energy as light are used in nuclear medicine both for imaging (see the description of scintillation crystals in the next chapter) and for recording cumulative radiation exposure.

Particles and photons from radioactive sources striking these crystals (Figure 4.16(a)) cause electrons (and positively charged holes) to be released from the atoms of the crystal (Figure 4.16(b)).

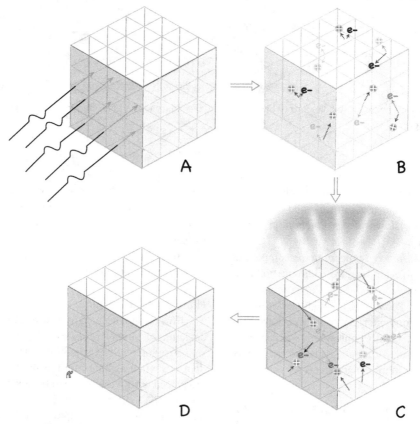

Figure 4.16 Luminescent crystal. (a) Photons strike crystal; (b) electrons and positively charged holes are released and then recombine (c), causing emission of light photons; (d) crystal returns to stable state.

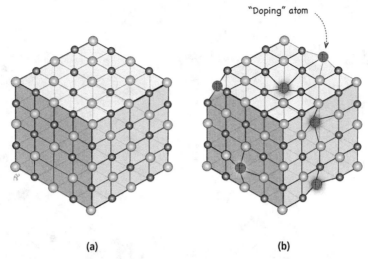

"Doping" atom

(a)   (b)

Figure 4.17 Luminescent crystal (a) without and (b) with "doping." Atoms used for doping are depicted as cross-hatched spheres.

These "excited" electrons contain excess energy. The excited electrons return to a stable state as they recombine with the positive holes, and in the process release their excess energy as light (Figure 4.16(c) and (d)).

Crystals that emit light as soon as they are exposed to radiation are useful for imaging, but not for recording cumulative radiation exposure. Fortunately, some luminescent crystals absorb energy from radiation but do not emit all of the absorbed energy immediately. A portion of the absorbed energy remains in the crystal until the crystal is exposed to another external energy source, such as heat or laser light. Usually, the absorptive properties of these crystals are improved by contaminating, or "doping," the crystal with small amounts of other elements (Figure 4.17).

The added atoms alter the crystalline structure such that the electrons and holes released by radiation exposure are prevented from returning to a stable state; the electrons and holes are "trapped" until external energy is applied to the "doped" crystal. This applied external energy alters the crystalline structure enough for the electrons and holes to escape their "traps" and return to a stable state. As they return to their stable state, they release the excess energy that was deposited by the initial radiation exposure (Figure 4.18).

Thermoluminescent detectors

Examples of crystalline substances that are commonly used to make thermoluminescent badges are calcium fluoride doped with manganese (CaF_2:Mn) and lithium fluoride doped with magnesium and titanium (LiF:Mg,Ti). When these badges are sent (usually after a period of one or more months) to an outside laboratory for reading, they are carefully exposed to heat (the "thermo" portion of "thermoluminescent"). The application of energy in the form of heat causes the release of the trapped electrons (and positive holes). As the electrons and holes return to their stable state, their excess "stored" energy is released as light. The amount of released light is proportional to the amount of energy stored in the crystal during its repeated exposures to radiation. Since, during the process of heating, the atomic configuration returns to a stable state, these badges can only be read once (however, once read, they are restored to their original state and can be reused).

Optically luminescent detectors

An example of a common crystalline substance that is used in optically luminescent detectors is aluminum oxide doped with carbon (Al_2O_3:C). Instead of heat, laser light (hence the term "optical")

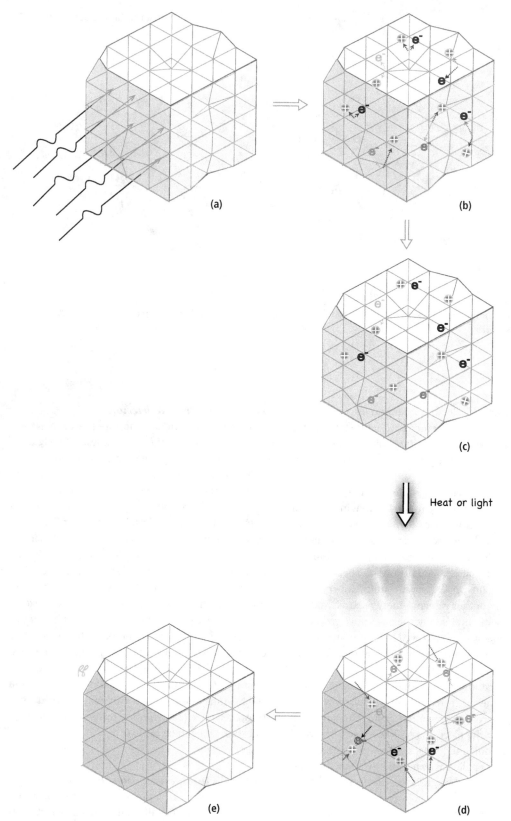

Heat or light

Figure 4.18 Thermoluminescent or optically luminescent crystal. (a) Photons strike crystal; (b) electrons and positively charged holes are released and remain trapped (c) until energy in the form of heat or laser light is applied, after which they recombine causing emission of light photons (d) and the crystal returns to a stable state (e).

is applied to these detector materials to release the electrons and positive holes from their "traps" in the doped crystal. As with thermoluminescent materials, the quantity of light emitted from the crystal as the electrons recombine with positive holes is proportional to the cumulative amount of radiation exposure of the crystal. The advantage of these crystalline detectors is that they can be re-read several times.

Badge dosimeters made from thermoluminescent or optically luminescent crystals (in a powder form, enclosed within plastic) also contain small squares of different types of attenuating materials, which are placed in front of the crystals much as strips of these materials are placed in front of the film in photographic film badges (see Figure 5.15). By comparing the amounts of light emitted from the portions of crystalline material behind each attenuator, some characterization of the types (alpha, beta, and gamma) of the initial radiation exposure can be done and the energy of each type can be estimated.

Questions

1. Rank the following major voltage regions for gas detectors from highest applied voltage to lowest applied voltage:
   (1) Ionization region.
   (2) Proportional region.
   (3) Geiger region.

2. True or false: Gas-filled detectors are highly efficient for the detection of high-energy gamma photons and X-rays as well as low-energy beta particles.

3. Which of the following radiation detectors are classified as ionization chambers?
   (1) Pen dosimeter.
   (2) Geiger counter.
   (3) Dose calibrator

4. True or false: Because of the near-maximal ionization of the gas molecules in a Geiger counter in response to each interaction of radiation with a gas molecule in the detector, Geiger counters cannot be used to distinguish between types or energies of radiation.

5. True or false: The film badge, unlike the pen dosimeter, can provide some information about the type and energy of the radiation an individual has received.

6. Which of the following are true about a dose calibrator?
   (1) It functions in the proportional region of voltage for gas chambers.
   (2) It is a type of ionization chamber.
   (3) It can be used to measure the activity of radionuclides because the current produced in the circuitry is proportional to the number of primary ionizations produced in the chamber by the nuclide.

7. True or false: The roentgen is a measure of radiation exposure in tissue.

8. Pocket dosimeters are useful because
   (1) They do not need charging.
   (2) They can differentiate between different types of radiation.
   (3) They can be used for immediate readings of radiation exposure.

9. True or false: Quenching gases are added to reduce the dead time between counts in gas amplification chambers such as the Geiger counter.

10. Which of the following are true about semiconductor materials?
    (1) For incoming radiation of the same energy, more ion pairs are created in a semiconductor than in air.
    (2) Semiconductors have more loosely bound outer-shell electrons than metals.
    (3) They are relatively expensive to produce.

11. Which of the following materials are currently used for measuring accumulated exposure for individuals working with radioactivity?
    (1) Gas detectors.
    (2) Film.
    (3) Optically luminescent detectors.
    (4) Geiger counters.
    (5) Thermoluminescent detectors.

Answers

1. High, Geiger; intermediate, proportional; low, ionization.

2. False. High-energy photons and X-rays will often pass through the detector without interacting with a gas molecule, and low-energy betas might not pass through the detection window.

3. (1), (3). All of the items listed are gas detectors, but only the pen dosimeter and the dose calibrator can be classified as ionization chambers. The Geiger counter, which functions in a higher voltage range than the ionization chambers, is better classified as a gas discharge device.

4. True.

5. True.

6. (2), (3).

7. False: It is a measure of radiation exposure in air only.

8. (3).

9. True.

10. (1) and (3). (2) is not correct, as semiconductors have fewer loosely bound outer-shell electrons than metals.

11. (2), (3), (5).

CHAPTER 5

Scintillation Detectors

Structure

Scintillation crystals

Scintillation is another term for luminescence, but applies specifically to light emission from crystals that are exposed to particles or photons from radiation. Scintillation crystals are translucent slabs in which gamma rays are converted to light. The most widely used crystals are made of sodium iodide (NaI); they are fragile and can easily be cracked. Because sodium iodide crystals absorb moisture from the atmosphere, they must be sealed in an airtight aluminum container.

Except at very low temperatures, pure sodium iodide crystals do not scintillate unless they are doped with small amounts (a fraction of a percent) of stable thallium (Tl). The thallium atoms dispersed in the crystal alter its response to the gamma ray photons and are said to "activate" the scintillation (Figure 5.1).

The process of converting gamma rays to light is complex, but it can be summarized as absorption of the gamma ray energy by the crystal, leaving its electrons in an excited state. The gamma photon transfers its energy in one or more Compton or photoelectric interactions in the crystal. Each of the energetic electrons produced by these gamma ray interactions distributes its energy, in turn, among electrons in the crystal, leaving them in an excited state. As these return to their original state, some of their energy is released as light photons (Figure 5.2). For each keV of gamma ray energy absorbed by the crystal, approximately 40 light photons are emitted. In a typical detector arrangement, photomultiplier tubes are optically coupled to scintillation crystals to detect these light photons. The design of the crystal affects its performance. The thickness of the sodium iodide crystals used ranges from less than a centimeter to several centimeters. Thicker crystals, by absorbing more of the original and scattered gamma rays, have a relatively high sensitivity, because almost all of the gamma ray energy reaching the crystal is absorbed (Figure 5.3). Thinner crystals have a lower sensitivity because more photons escape. For photons in the 140 keV range (^{99m}Tc), typical thicknesses range from 0.6 to 1.2 cm.

After the crystal has absorbed energy from a gamma ray impact, the excited electrons in the crystal do not all return to their original state at exactly the same time, but do so over the course of a few nanoseconds to milliseconds, depending on the scintillator. As a result, the light photons are also emitted by the crystal over a very short span of time instead of as a single simultaneous burst. Although we cannot perceive it, if one were to plot the amount of light released following a single gamma ray impact, it would appear as a curve instead of a sharp spike.

Photomultiplier tubes

The photomultiplier tube (PMT) is a vacuum tube with a **photocathode** on the end adjacent to the crystal. A photocathode is a light-sensitive material, usually a type of semiconductor. The PMT is coupled with a light-conductive transparent gel to the surface of the crystal (Figure 5.4). The transparent gel has the same refractive index as the crystal and the PMT window. The light striking the photocathode causes it to emit electrons, referred to as photoelectrons. On average, four to six light photons strike the photocathode for each photoelectron produced.

Essentials of Nuclear Medicine Physics and Instrumentation, Third Edition. Rachel A. Powsner, Matthew R. Palmer, and Edward R. Powsner.
© 2013 John Wiley & Sons, Ltd. Published 2013 by John Wiley & Sons, Ltd.

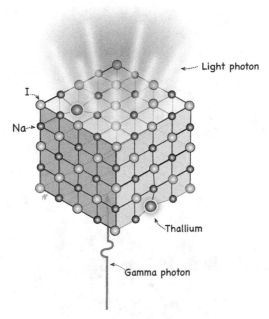

Figure 5.1 Scintillation crystal. A sodium iodide crystal "doped" with a thallium impurity is used to convert gamma photons into light photons.

The number of electrons produced at the photo-cathode is greatly increased by the multiplying action within the tube (Figure 5.5). As soon as they are produced, the electrons cascade along the multiplier portion of the tube, successively striking each of the tube's dynodes. These are metal electrodes, each held at a progressively higher voltage. As an electron strikes a dynode, it knocks out two to four new electrons, each of which joins the progressively larger pulse of electrons cascading toward the anode at the end of the tube. In other words, for each electron entering a cascade of just three such dynodes, there will be between 2^3 and 4^3 electrons leaving; cascading against 10 dynodes will yield between 2^{10} and 4^{10} electrons.

Preamplifiers and amplifiers

The current from the photomultiplier must be amplified further before it can be processed and counted. Despite the multiplication in the photomultiplier tube, the number of electrons yielded by the chain of events that begins with the absorption of a single gamma ray in the crystal is still small and must be increased further, or amplified. Typically, this amplification is a two-stage process.

In the first stage, a small preamplifier located close to the photomultiplier increases the number of charges sufficiently to allow a current to be transmitted through a cable to the main amplifier. In the second stage, the current of the electrical pulse is increased further by the main amplifier by as much as a thousandfold (see Figure 5.5).

Pulse-height analyzer

The amplifiers are designed to ensure that the amplitude of each pulse is proportional to the energy absorbed in the crystal from the gamma radiation. The amplitude of each electrical pulse from the amplifiers is measured in the electrical circuits of a **pulse-height analyzer**. A tally is kept, showing the number of pulses of each height. A plot of the number of pulses against their height—that is, their energy—is called a **pulse-height spectrum**.

The pulse-height analyzer is often used to "select" only those pulses (conventionally called Z-pulses) that correspond to a range of acceptable energies. This range is called the **energy window**. A window setting of 20% for the 140 keV photopeak of ^{99m}Tc means that Z-pulses corresponding to a 28 keV range centered on 140 keV (from 126 to 154 keV) will be accepted and counted (Figure 5.6).

The energy spectrum from a sodium iodide detector

The shape of the pulse-height spectrum is dependent on the photon energies and the characteristics of the crystal detector. We shall now review some of the general features of the spectrum, and examine the components of the spectrum obtained from an NaI crystal, the most commonly used crystal.

Calibrating the energy spectrum

The energy scale (horizontal axis) can be calibrated in absolute terms by using a radionuclide whose photon energy is well known, usually one with a simple decay scheme. The most prominent peak, seen as a high point in the spectrum, is then assigned the energy value corresponding to the known energy of the principal gamma ray of the radionuclide under observation.

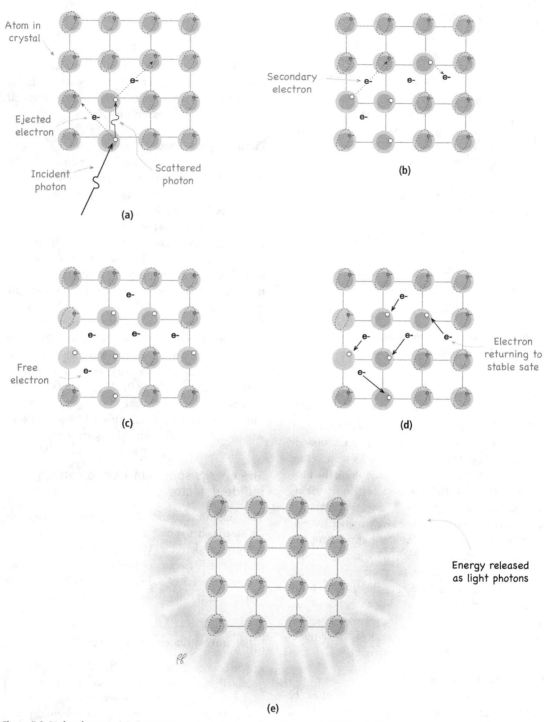

Figure 5.2 Light photons. (a) Gamma rays eject electrons from the crystal through Compton scattering and the photoelectric effect. (b, c) The ejected electrons, in turn, produce a large number of secondary electrons. (d, e) During de-excitation (oversimplified in this drawing), energy is released in the form of visible light.

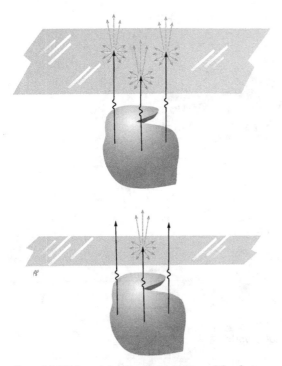

Figure 5.3 Thick crystals stop a larger fraction of the photons.

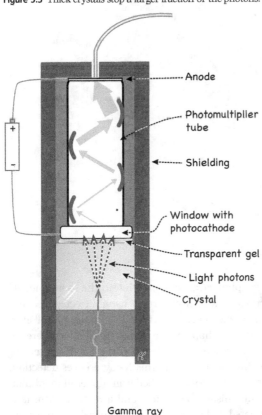

Figure 5.4 Sodium iodide crystal scintillation detector.

Photopeak

When a gamma photon deposits all of its energy in the crystal, the amplifier output is a single electrical pulse whose amplitude is, as discussed above, proportional to the energy of the original gamma photon. Ideally, this conversion of gamma energy to electrical pulse would be identical for each photon, and a plot of these pulses would appear as a single narrow "spike." However, owing mainly to the statistical variation in the number of visible-light photons produced upon interaction of the gamma ray with the scintillator, the plot of the electrical pulses corresponding to the photon energy is a blurred version of the original spike (Figure 5.7).

The photopeaks in the spectrum correspond to the principal energies of the gamma rays from the radioactive source. Figure 5.8 shows a typical spectrum, from a sample of ^{99m}Tc. The relatively sharp, prominent peak at 140 keV is called the photopeak. It is produced by the predominant gamma photon from the decay of ^{99m}Tc. The horizontal axis of the pulse-height spectrum represents the energy, typically in keV or MeV. The vertical axis represents the number of photons detected at each point on the energy scale.

Other peaks in the energy spectrum of the source

Several other important peaks—the Compton, iodine escape, annihilation, and coincidence peaks—are briefly discussed below.

Compton peak (or compton edge)

Compton scattering was introduced in Chapter 2. If both the **Compton electron** and the deflected photon are detected, their total energy will equal that of the incident photon, and the event will register in the photopeak. However, the scattered photon often escapes detection, so that the event leaves only the energy of the Compton electron in the crystal. These Compton electrons, whose energies are always less than that of the incident photon, register to the left of the photopeak.

The Compton electrons can have any energy from nearly zero up to a characteristic maximum called the Compton peak or edge. The value of the maximum energy can be calculated as follows:

$$E_{\text{maximum Compton electron}} = \frac{E^2_{\text{incident photon}}}{(E_{\text{incident photon}} + 256\text{ keV})}$$

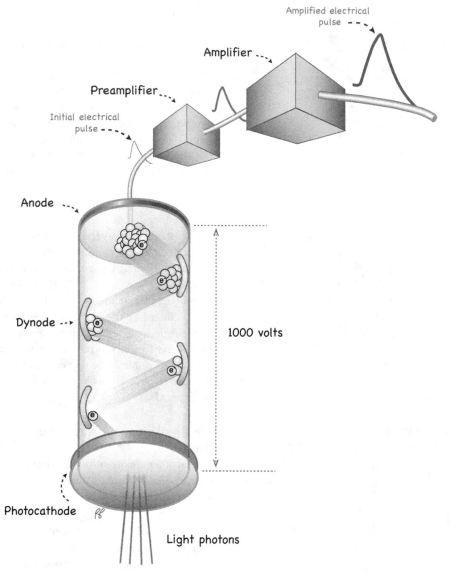

Figure 5.5 Photomultiplier tube and its preamplifier and amplifier.

For example, the maximum Compton electron energy for a ^{99m}Tc 140 keV photon is 50 keV. The Compton plateau refers to electron energies that are less than the Compton peak; the Compton valley reflects the sum of the energies of multiple Compton electrons generated by a single photon (see Figure 5.8).

Iodine escape peak

The photoelectric effect contributes indirectly to the existence of a small peak below the photopeak. When an incoming photon is absorbed as a result of a photoelectric interaction in the sodium iodide crystal, a K-shell electron is usually ejected. Because the K-shell vacancy is then filled by an L-shell electron (see Chapter 3), a 28 keV X-ray (the difference in binding energies between the L and K shells of iodine) is emitted. If this X-ray escapes detection, the total energy absorbed from the original photon is diminished by 28 keV, and a new, small peak is created 28 keV below the photopeak (Figure 5.9). This is called the **iodine escape peak**. It can only be seen as separate from the photopeak at relatively

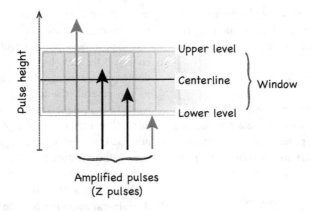

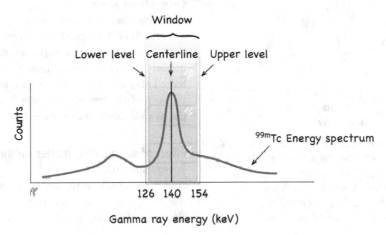

Figure 5.6 Pulse-height analyzer. The incoming pulse (Z-pulse) is proportional to the energy of the initial gamma ray photon. The pulse-height analyzer accepts only those that fall within the window (depicted as black arrows in top illustration).

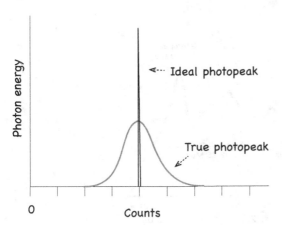

Figure 5.7 Imperfections in the crystal and circuitry cause blurring of the photopeak.

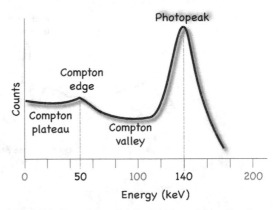

Figure 5.8 Compton peak (edge). (Adapted from Harris CC, Hamblen DP, Francis JE. Oak Ridge National Laboratory basic principles of scintillation counting for medical investigators. In: Ross DA (ed.) *Medical Gamma-ray Spectrometry*. Oak Ridge, TN: US Atomic Energy Commission, Division of Technical Information, 1959.)

low energies, where the spread of the photopeak is relatively small; at higher photopeak energies, the iodine escape peak is obscured by the spread of the photopeak.

Annihilation peak

If an entering photon is energetic enough (>1.02 MeV), it may be absorbed near the nucleus of an atom, creating a positron and an electron. This process is called **pair production**. The posi-

tron (β^+) will undergo annihilation with an electron, producing two 511 keV photons. In the same reaction, a new photon will be emitted with an energy 1.02 MeV less than that of the incident photon. If the energy of all three photons is detected by the crystal, the total absorbed energy will be equal to the original energy of the incident photon and will contribute to the photopeak. If, however, one 511 keV photon escapes the detector, the sum will be reduced by 511 keV; if both photons escape, the sum will be reduced by 1.02 MeV. The resulting peaks are called the **single-escape** and **double-escape annihilation peaks**, respectively (Figure 5.10).

Coincidence peak

Some nuclides emit two or more photons. Most often, each of these produces its own characteristic photopeak in the spectrum. However, if two photons impact the crystal simultaneously, the detector will record only a single event with an energy equal to the sum of the two photon energies. This result is the so-called **coincidence peak** (Figure 5.11).

Effect of surrounding matter on the energy spectrum

So far, we have considered the appearance of the energy spectrum for a point source in air. However, the daily practice of nuclear medicine

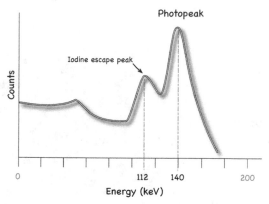

Figure 5.9 Iodine escape peak. (Adapted from Harris CC, Hamblen DP, Francis JE. Oak Ridge National Laboratory basic principles of scintillation counting for medical investigators. In: Ross DA (ed.) *Medical Gamma-ray Spectrometry*. Oak Ridge, TN: US Atomic Energy Commission, Division of Technical Information, 1959.)

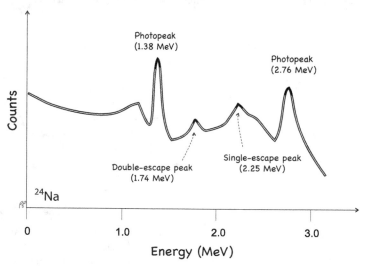

Figure 5.10 Annihilation peaks. (Adapted from Ross DA, Harris CC. *The Measurement of Clinical Radioactivity*, ORNL-4153. Oak Ridge, TN: Oak Ridge National Laboratory, 1968.)

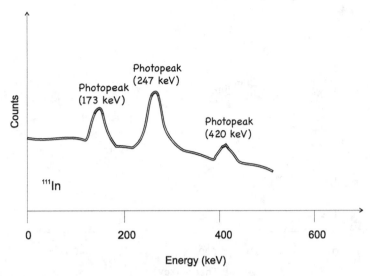

Figure 5.11 Coincidence peaks.

rarely involves imaging point sources in air with unshielded NaI(Tl) crystals. The lead used to shield the crystal and the water and tissue surrounding the radioactive source alter the shape of the energy spectrum.

Backscatter peak

When lead shielding surrounds the crystal, photons may exit the crystal without detection only to be deflected 180° off the lead back into the crystal. These photons account for the **backscatter peak**. Their energy is equal to

$$E_{\text{backscattered photon}} = \frac{E_{\text{incident photon}}}{(1 + E_{\text{incident photon}}/256 \text{ keV})}$$

Backscatter peaks are only evident when the incident energy is great enough to cause a significant degree of Compton scattering in lead (approximately 200 keV).

Characteristic lead X-ray peak

A photoelectric interaction in the lead shielding will result in ejection of a K-shell electron along with the prompt emission of an X-ray. The energy of this X-ray is 72 keV and is equal to the difference between the binding energies of the L and K shells of lead. The emitted X-ray can be detected by the

crystal and contributes to the **characteristic lead X-ray peak** at 72 keV.

Additional compton scattering from the medium surrounding the source

Many of the photons emitted by a source will undergo Compton scattering in surrounding water or tissue. As a consequence, there will be fewer counts in the photopeak. The Compton photons may be seen by the detector and add to the counts below the photopeak. The effects of water on the energy spectrum of ^{51}Cr can be seen in Figure 5.12.

Characteristics of scintillation detectors

Energy resolution

Because the peaks of an energy spectrum are not sharp spikes but are statistically broadened, the detector may not be able to separate peaks produced by photons of similar energy. The distance between the closest peaks that the detector can distinguish determines the energy resolution of the detector.

Decay time

Although scintillation detectors absorb incoming radiation virtually instantaneously, the emission of visible light takes place over an extended period of time. This brief interval is referred to as the **decay**

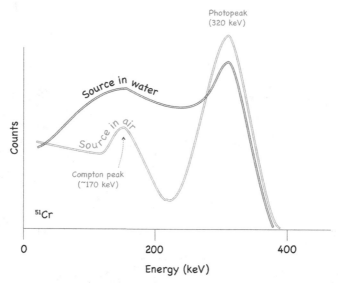

Figure 5.12 The effect of water on the ^{51}Cr energy spectrum. (Adapted from Harris CC, Hamblen DP, Francis JE. Oak Ridge National Laboratory basic principles of scintillation counting for medical investigators. In: Ross DA (ed.) *Medical Gamma-ray Spectrometry*. Oak Ridge, TN: US Atomic Energy Commission, Division of Technical Information, 1959.)

time of the crystal and is about 230 ns for NaI(Tl). If a second gamma photon enters the crystal during this time, it will add to the total output of the light pulse in a process referred to as **pulse pileup**. These events cannot be distinguished as separate detection events, and so the energy measured by the analyzer will be the sum of the two gamma energies.

Efficiency

The fundamental meaning of efficiency is the amount observed as a fraction of the amount expected. The **overall efficiency** of a detector can be considered in terms of **geometric** and **intrinsic** efficiency.

Overall efficiency

The ratio of the number of counts actually registered by the detector to the number of decays generated by a source in a given period of time is the **overall efficiency**. For a well detector, this is simply the number of counts recorded divided by the number of decays in the specimen. For a camera, it is the ratio of the number of counts within the image of the target organ, the so-called region of interest (ROI), to the number of decays of the radionuclide present in the organ. Overall efficiency can

be measured, or at least reasonably approximated, by counting a sample container filled with a known quantity of radioactivity.

Using this method, the efficiency is given by the ratio of the number of counts recorded (if one is using a well detector) or seen in the ROI (if one is using a camera) to the number of actual decays. Except for attenuation within the sample or its container, the number of decays in the specimen will be 10^6 decays per megabecquerel (MBq) or 3.7×10^4 decays per microcurie (μCi).

As a practical matter, the efficiency of modern detectors is not a consideration in the daily work of a nuclear medicine department. Not only are relatively high count rates available from patients and specimens, but also most quantitative work is based on comparison of count rates from a sample (such as a urine sample) with a standard (such as the standard used for a Schilling test) using the same device. Because the efficiency is the same for both standard and sample, the exact value of the efficiency is inconsequential. The detector efficiency is more important when the radioactivity in a wipe test is being measured. Wipe tests are performed by wiping a small absorbent pad over a countertop or other surface and measuring the pad for any radioactive contamination. Here it is necessary to determine whether the activity measured on an absolute scale is below a prescribed limit, for example, less than $37\,\text{Bq/cm}^2$ ($1\,\text{nCi/cm}^2$).

Geometric efficiency

The size and shape of the detector relative to the organ being imaged determine how much of the radiation emanating from the organ is actually "seen" by the face of the detector. Because radiation emanates in all directions, a detector receives only a fraction of the total. The fraction of radiation striking, or "seen" by, the face of the detector will obviously be less for a smaller crystal than for a larger one, and will decrease further the farther away the detector is placed from the source.

The **geometric efficiency** is the ratio of the number of photons striking the face of the detector to the number of photons emitted by the target organ, assuming no significant losses in the air between patient and detector. Because the measurement of the number of photons actually striking the face of the detector may be difficult, it is usually satisfactory to infer the geometric efficiency from a physical measurement of the area of the detector face and the distance between it and the target.

Intrinsic efficiency

The intrinsic efficiency, a component of the overall efficiency, is the ratio of the number of counts recorded by the system to the number of photons striking the face of the detector. The intrinsic efficiency can be calculated most easily if a known source emitting a known number of photons is placed directly against the face of the detector. In this arrangement, any effect of geometric factors is usually small enough to be ignored.

Types of scintillation-based detectors

Some commonly used scintillation-based detectors are described below. All contain a sodium iodide crystal coupled to a single photomultiplier tube. The output of the photomultiplier tube is then routed through the preamplifier, amplifier, and pulse-height analyzer, as described above.

Thyroid probe

The thyroid probe (Figure 5.13) is a crystal scintillation detector for measuring the radioactivity in a patient's thyroid gland. The detector is supported on a stand by an adjustable arm that permits placement of the detector against the patient's neck. A cylindrical or slightly conical extension of the shielding around the crystal limits the field of view to the region of the thyroid gland. For measuring ^{123}I or ^{99m}Tc uptake in the gland, the sodium iodide scintillation crystal need only be half a centimeter thick. Thicker crystals, up to 2 cm thick, are more efficient for higher-energy radionuclides, such as [131]I.

Well counter

The well counter (Figure 5.14) is a shielded crystal with a hole, the "well," drilled in the center to hold a specimen in a test tube or vial. In this arrangement,

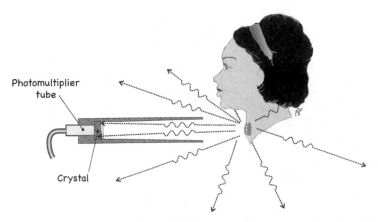

Figure 5.13 Thyroid probe. Shielded crystal scintillation detector, as used for measuring thyroid uptake.

Photomultiplier tube

Crystal

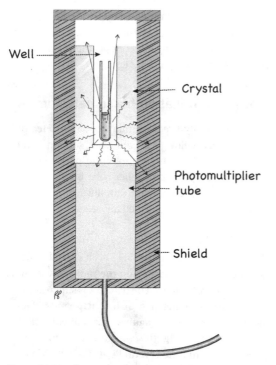

Well

Crystal

Photomultiplier tube

Shield

Figure 5.14 Well counter. Crystal scintillation detector constructed with an internal well for counting samples in vitro.

the specimen is surrounded by the crystal so that only a small fraction of the radiation escapes through the opening of the well. The size and thickness of the crystal are selected for efficient capture of photons. For radionuclides with low-energy emissions, the typical crystals used are cylinders 2–3 cm in diameter. Crystals two or three times larger are more efficient for higher energies such as those obtained from ^{131}I.

Dosimeters and area monitors

Scintillation detectors are available for use as dosimeters and handheld survey meters for the purpose of monitoring or searching for a source. Others are placed more permanently for area monitoring. In one commercial design, a series of detectors are arranged in a door-like frame through which personnel must pass before leaving a restricted area of a laboratory. The device is often equipped with an audible alarm to signal when the radiation is above an acceptable level.

Questions

1. Connect the following events with the corresponding components of a scintillation detector:
   (a) Photoelectrons are released in response to light photons.
   (b) Light photons are released in response to gamma photons.
   (c) The output of the photomultiplier tube is amplified to a more readily detectable level of current.
   (d) The multiplying action of successive steps yields a very large number of electrons in response to each photoelectron.
   (1) Photomultiplier tube.
   (2) Preamplifier.
   (3) Crystal.
   (4) Photocathode surface of photomultiplier tube.

2. Name the following features that can be seen in the energy spectrum obtained from a sodium iodide crystal detector:
   (a) Can be seen at 28 keV below the photopeak.
   (b) Energy of photon source.
   (c) Can be seen at 511 and 1020 keV below the photopeak of the high-energy photon.
   (d) Peak near 420 keV emitted by a ^{111}In source.
   (e) Maximum Compton electron energy.
   (f) 72 keV.
   (1) Photopeak.
   (2) Compton peak or edge.
   (3) Annihilation peaks.
   (4) Iodine escape peak.
   (5) Coincidence peak.
   (6) Lead X-ray peak.
   (7) Backscatter peak.

3. True or false: A detector that can distinguish separate photopeaks at 200 and 205 keV has a better energy resolution than a detector that can only distinguish photopeaks as close as 200 and 250 keV.

4. Match each of the listed terms (1)–(3) below to one of the following definitions:
   (a) Electrical output from the preamplifier and amplifier connected to a photomultiplier tube in response to a photon interaction in the crystal.
   (b) Range of acceptable photon energies.
   (c) Used to select Z-pulses within the upper and lower limits of the energy window.
   (1) Pulse height analyzer.
   (2) Energy window.
   (3) Z-pulse.

5. A single 15% energy window is set symmetrically on the 159 keV photopeak for an iodine-123 imaging study in a gamma camera. The lower and upper energy windows are:
   (a) 0 and 159 keV.
   (b) 159 and 183 keV.
   (c) 143 and 175 keV.
   (d) 147 and 171 keV.
   (e) 135 and 159 keV.

6. Scintillation detectors convert:
   (a) Gamma ray energy into a current.
   (b) Visible light into ultraviolet light.
   (c) Gamma ray energy into visible light.
   (d) Electron energy into potential energy.
   (e) Voltage into current.

7. Photomultiplier tubes:
   (a) Convert visible light into electrons that are then accelerated to provide amplification.
   (b) Convert electrons into dynodes that are then accelerated to provide amplification.
   (c) Detect the presence of ion pairs and produce a voltage pulse proportional to energy.
   (d) Are no longer used in nuclear imaging now that all-digital systems are preferred.

Answers

1. (a) (4). (b) (3). (c) (2). (d) (1).
2. (a) (4). (b) (1). (c) (3). (d) (5). (e) (2). (f) (6).
3. True.
4. (a) (3). (b) (2). (c) (1).

5. (d).
6. (c).
7. (a).

CHAPTER 6

Imaging Instrumentation

Theory and structure

The daily workload in a nuclear medicine department consists of "functional" imaging of organs, including the thyroid, brain, heart, liver, and kidneys. This is accomplished using a large scintillation device. In the 1950s, Harold Anger developed the basic design of the modern nuclear medicine camera. The **Anger camera** was a significant improvement over its predecessor, the rectilinear scanner. The components of the Anger camera are depicted in Figure 6.1.

Components of the imaging system

The following components of the imaging system are described in the order they are encountered by the gamma ray photons emitted from the patient's body.

Collimators

A collimator restricts the rays from the source so that each point in the image corresponds to a unique point in the source. Collimators are composed of thousands of precisely aligned **holes** (channels), which are formed by either casting hot lead or folding lead foil. They are usually depicted in cross section (Figure 6.2). Nuclides emit gamma ray photons in all directions. The collimator allows only those photons traveling directly along the long axis of each hole to reach the crystal. Photons emitted in any other direction are absorbed by the **septa** between the holes (Figure 6.3). Without a collimator in front of the crystal, the image would be indistinct (Figure 6.4).

There are several types of collimators, designed to channel photons of different energies. By an appropriate choice of collimator, it is possible to magnify or minify images, and to select between imaging quality and imaging speed.

Parallel-hole collimators

Low-energy all-purpose (LEAP) collimators: These collimators have relatively large holes, which allow the passage of many of the photons emanating from the patient. As such, they have relatively high sensitivity at the expense of resolution. Because the holes are larger, photons arising from a larger region of the source are accepted. As a result, image resolution is decreased (Figure 6.5, top image). The sensitivity of one such collimator has been calculated at approximately 500,000 cpm for a 1 µCi source, and the resolution is 1.0 cm at 10 cm from the surface of the collimator (Nuclear Fields Precision Microcast Collimators, Nuclear Fields B.V., The Netherlands; 140 keV ^{99m}Tc source). These collimators are useful for imaging low-energy photons such as those from ^{201}Tl, for which thick septa are not necessary. In addition, because of their moderately high sensitivity (resulting from thinner septa and bigger holes), they are advantageous for images of short duration such as sequential one-per-second images for a renal flow study. These collimators are sometimes called "GAP," or "general all-purpose," collimators.

> ### Distinction
>
> Nuclear medicine imaging systems are called cameras; just as standard cameras image light, these cameras image photons generated by nuclides. Unlike an X-ray machine, which creates photons (X-rays) that penetrate the body and detects those that emerge on the other side of the patient, nuclear medicine cameras utilize gamma photons from radiopharmaceuticals within the patient.

Essentials of Nuclear Medicine Physics and Instrumentation, Third Edition. Rachel A. Powsner, Matthew R. Palmer, and Edward R. Powsner.
© 2013 John Wiley & Sons, Ltd. Published 2013 by John Wiley & Sons, Ltd.

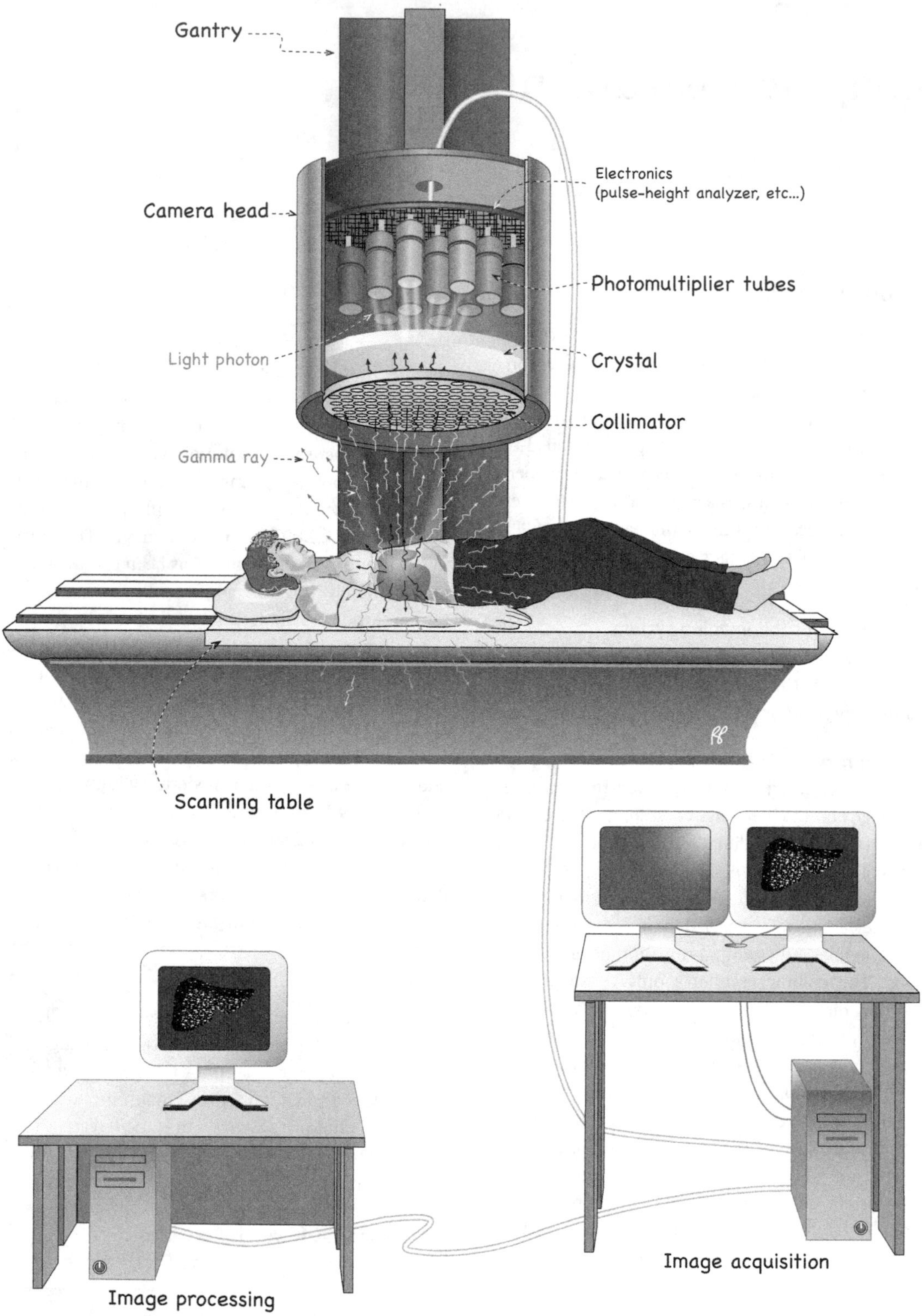

Figure 6.1 Components of a standard nuclear medicine imaging system.

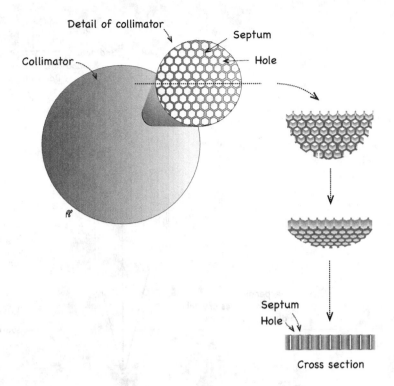

Figure 6.2 Collimator detail.

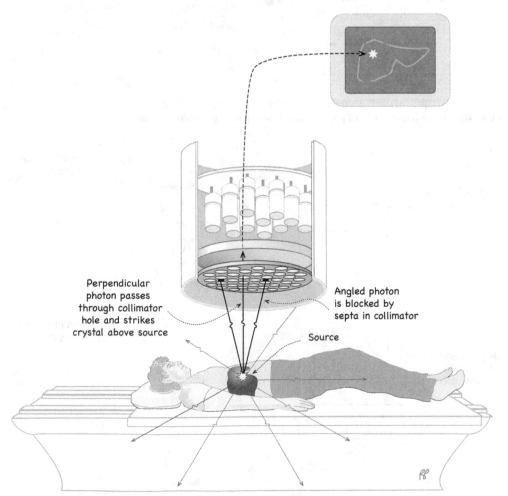

Figure 6.3 A collimator selects photons perpendicular to the plane of the collimator face.

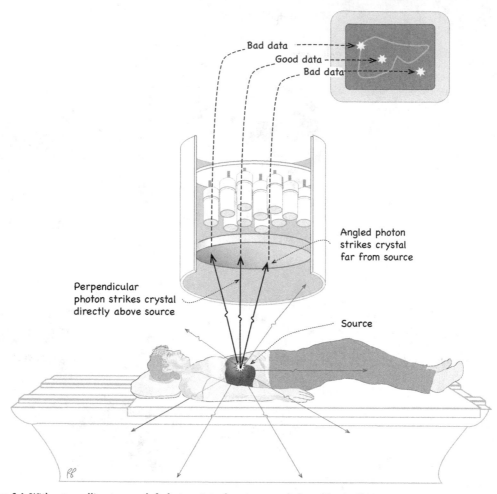

Figure 6.4 Without a collimator, angled photons introduce improperly located scintillations.

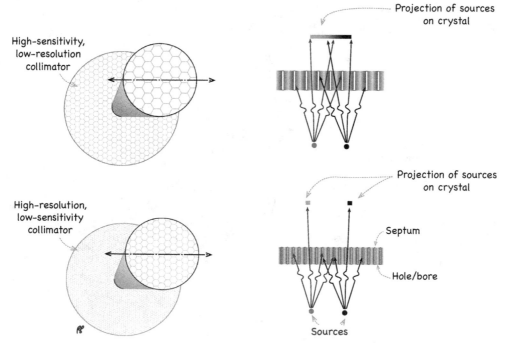

Figure 6.5 For the same bore length, the smaller the diameter, the higher the resolution.

High-resolution collimators: These collimators provide higher-resolution images than the LEAP collimators. They have more holes, which are both smaller in diameter and longer in length. The calculated sensitivity of one representative high-resolution collimator is approximately 185,000 cpm for a 0.037 MBq (1 µCi) source, and its nominal resolution is 0.65 cm at 10 cm from the face of the collimator (Nuclear Fields B.V.).

To compare the performance of a LEAP with a high-resolution collimator, let us look at the photons from two radioactive points in a liver. The photons from each of the points are emitted in all directions, but the detector can "see" only those photons that pass through the holes of the collimator. The relatively large holes in the LEAP collimator will also admit photons scattered at relatively large angles from the direct line between the liver and the crystal. This lowers the resolution because the angled photons have the effect of merging the images of two closely adjacent points (Figure 6.5). At the same time, the larger holes and correspondingly thinner septa give the LEAP collimator a higher sensitivity by admitting a higher percentage of the photons. The high-resolution collimator, on the other hand, admits photons from a smaller fraction of the organ, because more of its face is blocked by septa. In a reciprocal way, the narrower (see Figure 6.5) and/ or longer (Figure 6.6) bore of its holes better collimate those photons that do enter the collimator. As a result, relatively closely spaced details in the source are more likely to appear clearly separated in the image.

Sensitivity

"Sensitivity" refers to the ability of an imaging camera to detect the photons generated by the nuclides used. A **low-sensitivity** system detects a smaller number of the generated photons; a **high-sensitivity** system detects a greater number. For a given crystal, increasing the area occupied by holes as opposed to septa increases sensitivity. As a practical matter, this means larger holes and thinner septa. Another technique to improve sensitivity is to increase the thickness or area of the crystal.

Resolution

"Resolution" refers to the ability of a camera to distinguish between adjacent points in an organ, permitting detection of finer detail. The higher the resolution, the closer together are the points that can be distinguished. Using longer and/or narrower-bore holes increases resolution. A collimator's resolution is determined by its **angle of acceptance**. Only photons falling within the angle of acceptance can reach the crystal (Figure 6.7).

There is a trade-off between sensitivity and resolution. A high-sensitivity system has a relatively low resolution. To understand this, remember that although bigger holes admit more photons (higher sensitivity), they reduce the resolution (larger angle of acceptance).

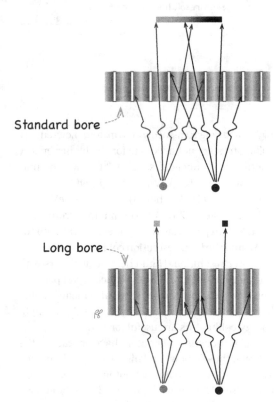

Standard bore

Long bore

Figure 6.6 For the same hole diameter, the longer the bore, the higher the resolution.

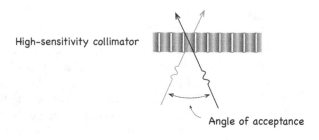

High-sensitivity collimator

Angle of acceptance

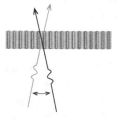

High resolution: narrower holes (bores)

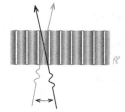

High resolution: longer bores

Figure 6.7 Angle of acceptance.

High- and medium-energy collimators: Low-energy collimators are not adequate for the higher-energy photons from nuclides such as ^{67}Ga (which emits 394, 300, and 185 keV photons, in addition to its low-energy 93 keV photon), ^{131}I (376 keV), and ^{111}In (245 and 173 keV). The photons from these nuclides can penetrate the thinner septa of both the LEAP and the high-resolution collimators, resulting in poorer resolution. High-energy collimators with thicker septa (Figure 6.8) to reduce septal penetration are used, but thicker septa also mean smaller holes and, consequently, lower sensitivity. High-energy collimators are useful for ^{131}I.

Medium-energy collimators have characteristics between those of low- and high-energy collimators. They can be used to image photons emitted by ^{67}Ga and ^{111}In. The terms high-, medium-, and low-energy are not rigidly defined, and usage may vary from institution to institution.

Slant-hole collimators: These are parallel-hole collimators with holes directed at an angle to the surface of the collimator. The slant-hole collimator provides an oblique view for better visualization of an organ that would otherwise be obscured by an overlying structure while permitting the face of the collimator to remain close to the body surface (Figure 6.9).

Nonparallel-hole collimators: Nonparallel-hole collimators provide a wider or narrower field of view. The cone-like pattern of holes allows these collimators to enlarge or reduce the size of the image.

Converging and diverging collimators: A parallel-hole collimator and an image formed with it are shown in Figure 6.10. At least for this simple example, the organ and the image are the same size. In a converging collimator, however, the holes are not parallel but are angled inward, toward the organ, as

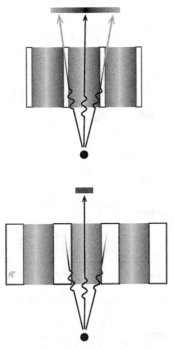

Figure 6.8 Thicker septa are used to block high- and medium-energy photons.

shown in Figure 6.11. Consequently, the organ appears larger at the face of the crystal.

Diverging collimators achieve a wider field of view by angling the holes the opposite way, outward toward the organ. This is used most often on cameras with a small crystal, such as a portable camera. Using a diverging collimator, a large organ such as the lung can be captured on the face of a smaller crystal (Figure 6.12).

Memory hint

Remembering the difference between diverging and converging collimators is easier if you realize that in the former the holes diverge (or spread out) toward the patient, whereas in the latter they converge (come together) toward the patient.

Pinhole collimators: These have a single hole—the pinhole—usually 2–4 mm in diameter. Like a camera lens, the pinhole projects the image upside down and reversed right to left at the crystal (Figure

6.13). The image is usually corrected electronically on the viewing screen. A pinhole collimator can be used to generate magnified images of a small organ such as the thyroid or a joint.

Fan beam collimators: These are a cross between a converging and a parallel-hole collimator. They are designed for use on cameras with rectangular heads when smaller organs such as the brain and heart are being imaged. When viewed from one direction (along the short dimension of the rectangle), the holes are parallel. When viewed from the other direction (along the long dimension of the rectangle), the holes converge (Figure 6.14). This arrangement allows the data from the patient to be spread to better fill the surface of the crystal.

Camera head

The camera head contains the crystal, photomultiplier tubes (PMTs), and associated electronics (see Figure 6.1). The **head housing** envelopes and shields these internal components. Typically, it includes a thin layer of lead. A **gantry** supports the heavy camera head.

Crystals, photomultiplier tubes, preamplifiers, and amplifiers: The crystal for an imaging camera is a large slab of thallium-"doped" NaI crystal similar to that used for the scintillation probes described in Chapter 5. It should be noted that the thickness of a crystal affects its resolution as well as its sensitivity. Although thicker crystals have higher sensitivity, the resolution is lower because gamma rays may be scattered and absorbed farther from the point at which they entered the crystal (Figure 6.15). Sixty or more PMTs may be attached to the back surface of the crystal using light-conductive jelly. Each of these functions very much like the single PMT described in Chapter 5. The preamplifiers and amplifier are also discussed there.

Positioning algorithm: The amount of light received by a photomultiplier tube is related to the proximity of the tube to the site of interaction of the gamma ray in the crystal. The PMT closest to the site of interaction receives the greatest number of photons and generates the greatest output pulse; the tube farthest from the nuclide source receives the fewest light photons and generates the smallest pulse.

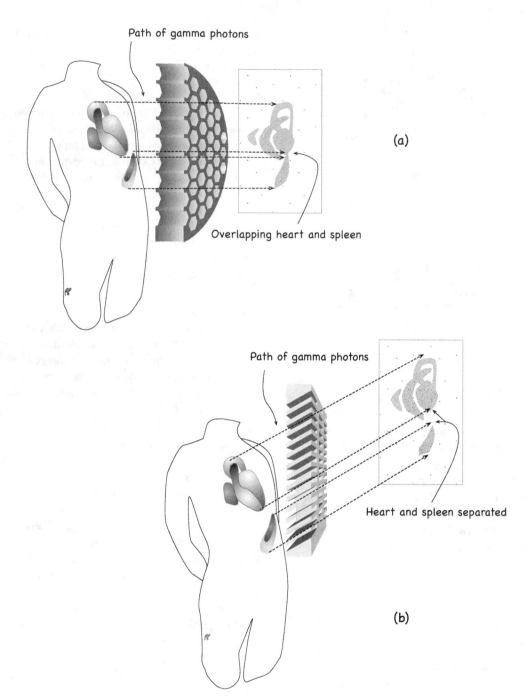

Figure 6.9 (a) Parallel-hole and (b) slant-hole collimators.

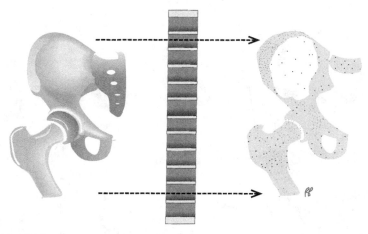

Figure 6.10 Parallel-hole collimator.

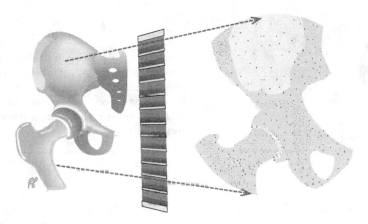

Figure 6.11 Converging collimator.

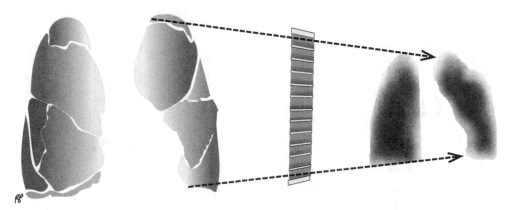

Figure 6.12 Diverging collimator.

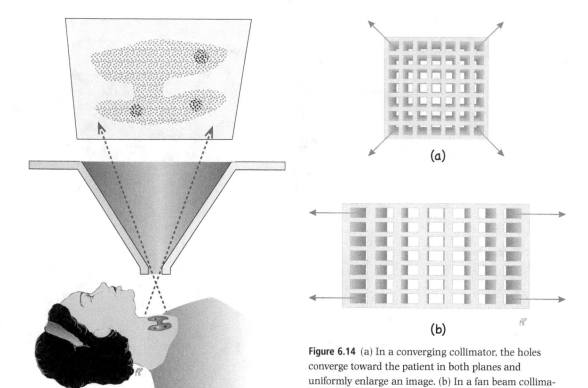

Figure 6.13 Pinhole collimator.

Figure 6.14 (a) In a converging collimator, the holes converge toward the patient in both planes and uniformly enlarge an image. (b) In a fan beam collimator, the holes converge in one plane but are parallel in the other. The arrows demonstrate the paths of photons coming from the patient.

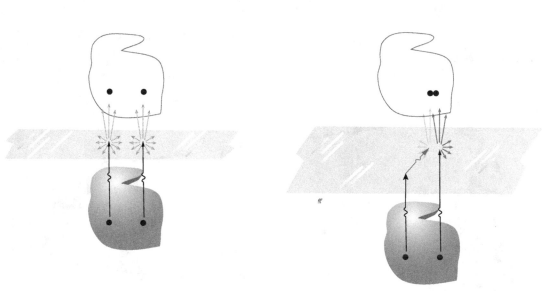

Figure 6.15 Scattering of photons in a thicker crystal reduces resolution.

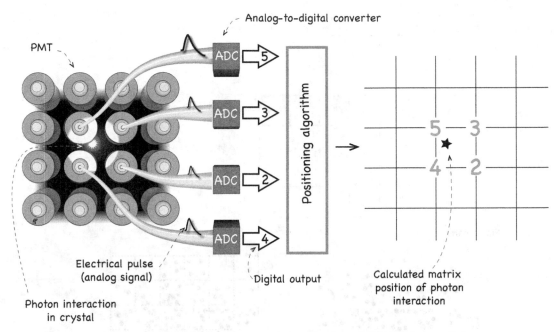

Figure 6.16 The positioning algorithm improves image resolution. The closer the PMT to the site of photon interaction in the crystal, the greater the analog signal output (current pulse). This signal is converted to a digital value by the analog-to-digital converters, and this digital value is used to calculate the corresponding matrix position of the photon interaction in the image stored on the computer.

Although an image can be formed solely from the points corresponding to the PMT with the highest output at each photon interaction, the number of resolvable points is then limited to the total number of PMTs (up to 128 per camera).

A **positioning algorithm** improves the resolution by combining signals from adjacent tubes (Figure 6.16). The electrical pulse generated by each PMT is first digitized by an analog-to-digital converter (ADC). These digital values are then transmitted to the positioning algorithm, which is a part of the computer-processing equipment in the camera head. Since the computer or positioning algorithm "knows" the location of each PMT on the surface of the crystal, it can estimate the site of the gamma ray interaction in the crystal by "weighing-in" the digital value of the amount of light each PMT receives.

Pulse-height analyzer: The function of the pulse-height analyzer was discussed in the preceding chapter (see Figure 5.6). Following each gamma photon interaction in the crystal, the sum of the digital outputs from all of the PMTs is proportional to the energy of the gamma photon striking the crystal. This summed output is called the **Z-pulse**. The pulse-height analyzer accepts only those Z-pulses that correspond to the gamma energy of interest. Each accepted Z-pulse and its location (as determined by the positioning algorithm) are stored in the computer.

Persistence scope

In the past, a persistence scope was made with a phosphor that faded very slowly to provide a slowly changing view of the x, y locations of the Z-pulses that were accepted (each of which corresponded to the location of a gamma ray). At present, the same result is achieved with much greater flexibility by storing the image in computer memory and using it to update the image on the screen slowly or rapidly. This allows the person who is acquiring the scan to adjust the position of the patient prior to recording the final image on film or computer.

Computers

Nuclear medicine computers are used for the acquisition, storage, and processing of data. The image data are stored in digital form (**digitized**) as follows: For each Z-pulse that is accepted by the pulse-height

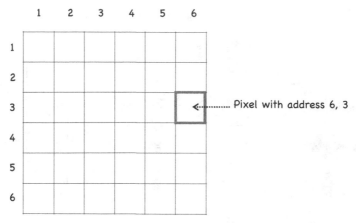

Figure 6.17 Small matrix.

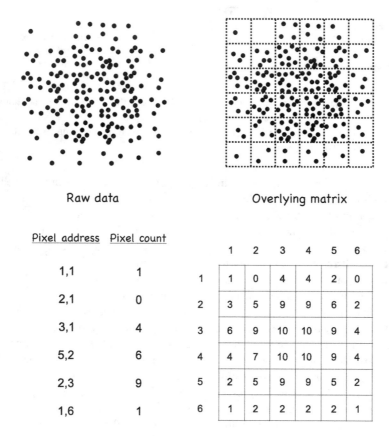

Figure 6.18 Storing image data in a matrix.

analyzer, one count is added to the storage location that corresponds to its x, y location determined by the positioning circuit. The data storage can be visualized as a **matrix**, a kind of two-dimensional checkerboard. Each position in the matrix corre-

sponds to a **pixel**, which has a unique "address" composed of the row and column of its location (Figure 6.17). Data are digitized by assigning a matrix position to every accepted photon (Figure 6.18). Matrices are defined by the number of subdivisions along each axis. The operator can select from several matrix configurations with successively finer divisions: 64×64, 128×128, 256×256, and 512×512, or more. These numbers refer to the number of columns and rows in these square matrices. Note that the outside dimensions of all of these matrices are the same size; what varies is the pixel size and hence the total number of pixels. A 64×64 matrix has 4096 pixels, a 128×128 matrix has 16,384 pixels, and so on.

The greater the number of pixels, the smaller is each pixel for a given field of view, and the better preserved is the resolution of the image (Figure 6.19). The camera and computer system cannot reliably distinguish between two points that are separated by less than one pixel. In Figure 6.20,

three "hot spots" are seen in the kidney parenchyma. With the coarser matrix (larger pixel size) depicted in the upper portion of the figure, two of the three spots are in a single pixel. In the finer matrix pictured in the lower portion, all three points are distinct, as there are now several "cold" pixels between the "hot" pixels.

The size of a pixel is inversely related to the dimensions of the matrix for a given field of view. For a 32 cm camera field of view mapped onto a 64×64 computer matrix, each pixel will measure 0.5 cm on a side. For the same camera, each pixel of a 128×128 matrix will measure 0.25 cm on a side. Similarly, a 256×256 matrix will divide the field of view into pixels measuring 0.125 cm on a side. This means that points that are closer to each

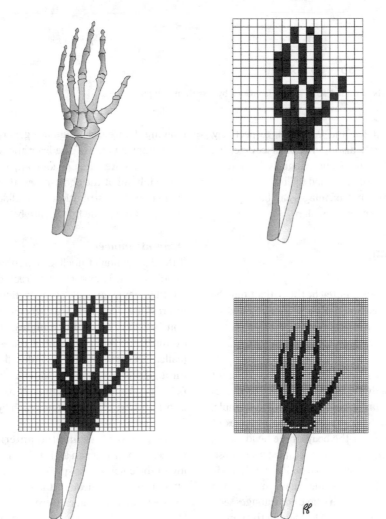

Figure 6.19 Effect of matrix configuration on image resolution.

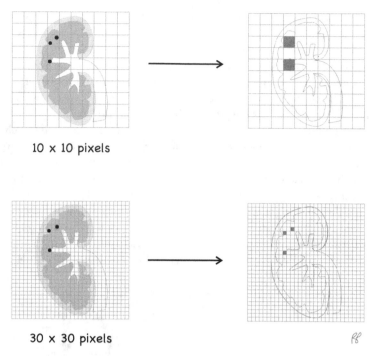

10 × 10 pixels

30 × 30 pixels

Figure 6.20 A matrix cannot resolve points separated by less than one pixel.

other than 0.5, 0.25, and 0.125 cm, respectively, cannot be separately distinguished. Of course, the maximum resolution of the image is limited by the resolution of the camera and collimator. Once the data are stored in a matrix, images can be displayed on the computer screen or on film.

Planar imaging

Image acquisition

The gamma photons emitted by the patient may be acquired in various forms: static, dynamic, gated, or planar tomographic images.

Static images

Static imaging is used to collect images of different regions of the body or differently angled (oblique) views of a particular region of interest. For example, a bone scan may be composed of static images of 12 different regions of the body (three head views, left arm, right arm, anterior chest, posterior chest, and so on) or anterior and posterior whole body images with additional static views of selected regions of the skeleton. The whole body images seen in Figure 6.21 were obtained by moving the gantry at a steady rate of 12 cm/min while acquiring the

imaging data. Liver scans are generally composed of six angled views of the liver and spleen; thyroid scans may have three or four angled views of the thyroid. In all of the above cases, there is very little change in the distribution of nuclide in the organ of interest while the images are being acquired.

Dynamic images

If the distribution of nuclide in an organ is changing rapidly and it is important to record this change, multiple rapid images of a particular region of interest are acquired. This type of image acquisition is called **dynamic imaging**. It is used, for example, to collect sequential one-second images (called **frames**) of the vascular flow of nuclide through the kidney. In the example shown in Figure 6.22, 60 frames were summed, or **compressed**, into 15 frames of four seconds each by adding every four frames together.

In Figure 6.23, sequential anterior abdominal images demonstrate an active bleeding site originating in the colon at the splenic flexure. Radiolabeled blood progresses through the descending colon to the rectum. The images were first acquired as 96 frames of 30 s duration. These images were then compressed into 16 images of three minutes each.

Dynamic imaging can be thought of as a type of video recording to "catch" images of fast action; static images are similar to photographs.

Gated images

Gated images are a variation of dynamic images, where continuous images are obtained of a moving organ (generally the heart), and the data are coordinated with the rate of movement (using electrocardiographic leads to keep track of the R–R interval for heart imaging). Gating is used to divide the emission data from the radioactive blood pool in a gated blood pool study (GBPS) or multigated acquisition (MUGA) into "frames" so that wall motion can be evaluated and the left ventricular ejection fraction can be calculated. During gated imaging, each cardiac cycle (the interval between R waves on the electrocardiogram) is divided into frames (Figure 6.24). The output of the electrocardiogram (attached to the patient) is connected to the nuclear medicine camera and computer. Each R wave "triggers" the collection of a set of frames. In this simplified example, the camera/computer combination is programmed to collect eight frames of 0.125 s each. This assumes that each heart beat is of one second's duration. Images of the cardiac blood pool collected from approximately 600 cardiac cycles are summed to create a single composite gated cycle image.

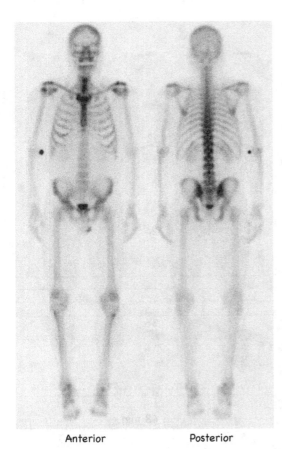

Anterior   Posterior

Figure 6.21 Bone scan.

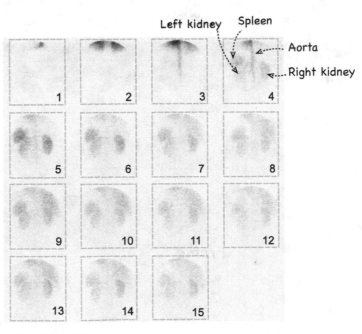

Figure 6.22 Sixty-second renal flow study.

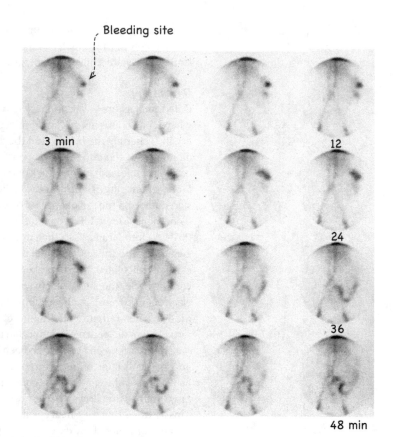

Figure 6.23 Gastrointestinal bleeding scan.

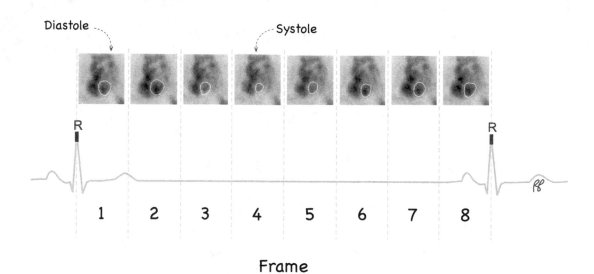

Figure 6.24 Gated blood pool study.

Questions

1. True or false: A parallel-hole collimator providing both high sensitivity and high resolution is difficult to design, principally because the requirements for sensitivity conflict with those for resolution.

2. Starting with a standard low-energy all-purpose collimator, what will happen to the images if you alter the collimator design by (an answer can be used more than once):
   (a) Lengthening the bores?
   (b) Increasing the number of holes while decreasing the size of each hole?
   (c) Thickening the septa?
       (i)   Higher resolution, lower sensitivity.
       (ii) Less septal penetration with higher-energy photons.
       (iii) Lower resolution, higher sensitivity.

3. True or false: In a converging-hole collimator, the holes angle inward toward the organ to be imaged. In consequence, the organ appears larger at the face of the crystal.

4. How many pixels of data can be stored in a 64×64 image matrix? Choose one of the following:
   (a) 128.
   (b) 256.
   (c) 512.
   (d) 1024.
   (e) 2048.
   (f) 4096.

5. The usual gamma camera head contains all of the following elements except:
   (a) Crystal.
   (b) Photomultiplier tubes.
   (c) Collimator.
   (d) Positioning circuit.
   (e) Pulse-height analyzer.
   (f) Focusing assembly.

6. Match the part of the imaging system with its function:
   (a) Positioning algorithm.
   (b) Photomultiplier tube.
   (c) Crystal.
   (d) Collimator
   (e) Gantry.
   (f) Pulse-height analyzer.
       (i)   Converts photon energy to light energy.
       (ii) Supports the camera head(s).
       (iii) Converts light energy to a small electrical pulse.
       (iv) Improves image resolution by factoring in the output of each PMT to better localize the position of the photon interaction in the imaging field.
       (v)   Accepts summed PMT output (Z-pulses) that correspond to the photon energy of the source.
       (vi) Restricts photon entry to the crystal so that each point in the image corresponds to a unique point in the source.

7. What is the pixel size for an image acquired with a field of view of size $32\,\text{cm} \times 32\,\text{cm}$ and a matrix of size 128×128?

Answers

1. True. For example, design for high sensitivity calls for large holes with thin septa, whereas high resolution calls for small holes and thick septa.
2. (a) (i). (b) (i). (c) (ii).
3. True.
4. (f) (4096) In a square matrix, $64 \times 64 = 4096$.
5. (f) (focusing assembly). This is an undefined term.
6. (a) (iv). (b) (iii). (c) (i). (d) (vi). (e) (ii). (f) (v).
7. $2.5 \times 2.5\,mm$ ($320\,mm/128 = 2.5\,mm$).

CHAPTER 7

Single-photon Emission Computed Tomography

Single-photon emission computed tomography (SPECT) cameras acquire multiple planar views of the radioactivity in an organ. The data are then processed mathematically to create cross-sectional views of the organ. SPECT utilizes the single photons emitted by gamma-emitting radionuclides such as ^{99m}Tc, ^{111}In, and ^{123}I. This is in contrast to positron emission tomography (PET), which utilizes the paired 511 keV photons arising from positron annihilation. PET is the subject of Chapter 8.

Equipment

Types of cameras

The simplest camera design for SPECT imaging is similar to that of a planar camera but with two additional features. First, the SPECT camera is constructed so that the head can rotate about the patient to acquire multiple views (Figure 7.1). Second, it is equipped with a computer that integrates the multiple images to produce the cross-sectional views of the organ.

To increase overall efficiency, most SPECT cameras are manufactured with more than one head—two being the most common number. The heads are mechanically rotated around the patient to obtain the multiple projection views (Figure 7.2). Recently, a number of dedicated cardiac SPECT cameras have come onto the market and gained wide acceptance; these will be discussed briefly at the conclusion of this chapter.

Angle of rotation of heads

Single-headed cameras must rotate a full 360° to obtain all necessary views of most organs. In con-

trast, each head of a double-headed camera need rotate only half as far, 180°, and each head of a triple-headed camera only 120° to obtain the same views. The cost of the additional heads must be balanced against the benefits of increased speed of acquisition.

Two-headed cameras: fixed and adjustable

Two-headed cameras can have a fixed, parallel configuration, a fixed, perpendicular configuration, or adjustable heads (Figure 7.3). Fixed, parallel heads (opposing heads) can be used for simultaneous anterior and posterior planar imaging or can be rotated as a unit for SPECT acquisition. Fixed, perpendicular heads, in an L-shaped unit, are used almost exclusively for cardiac and brain SPECT imaging.

Adjustable heads allow positioning of the heads in different angular configurations. The movable head can be moved closer to or farther along the ring from the other head so that the two heads are parallel (opposing), perpendicular (L-shaped), or separated by an intermediate angle. Thus the adjustable two-headed camera can be used for planar imaging and for large- and small-organ tomography.

Tomography

Tomos is the Greek word for "cut" or "section." "Tomography" is a name originally used for conventional X-ray systems that were modified to bring only a single plane through the patient into focus.

Essentials of Nuclear Medicine Physics and Instrumentation, Third Edition. Rachel A. Powsner, Matthew R. Palmer, and Edward R. Powsner.
© 2013 John Wiley & Sons, Ltd. Published 2013 by John Wiley & Sons, Ltd.

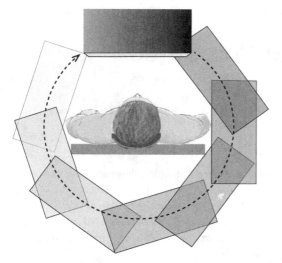

Figure 7.1 SPECT camera.

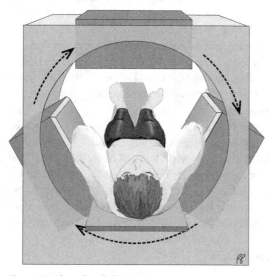

Figure 7.2 Three-headed SPECT camera.

Acquisition

The numerous sequential planar views acquired during tomographic acquisition are called **projection views**. They are little more than an intermediate step toward creating slices. Figure 7.4 shows an entire set of projection views that could be used to construct tomographic images of the liver and spleen. Because of the large number, 64 in this case, compared with the five typically used for a conventional liver–spleen scan (Figure 7.5), these projection views are most useful when displayed as a moderately rapid sequential presentation, the so-called **cine** view. The term "cine" is used because of its resemblance to movies.

Arc of acquisition

Tomographic projection views are most often acquired over an arc of 360° or 180°. A 360° arc of rotation of the camera heads is regularly used for most organs. A 180° arc is used for organs that are positioned on one side of the body, such as the heart.

Views of the heart are obtained in a 180° arc extending from the right anterior oblique position to the left posterior oblique position. The data from this 180° arc are considered adequate because photons exiting the body from the right posterior and lateral chest travel through more tissue and suffer greater attenuation than those exiting through the left side (Figure 7.6).

Number of projection tomographic views

Over a full 360° arc, 64 or 128 tomographic projections are usually collected; similarly, 32 or 64 views are generally obtained over a 180° arc.

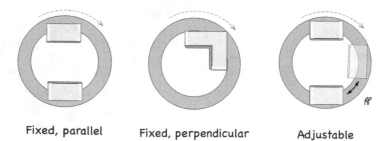

Fixed, parallel   Fixed, perpendicular   Adjustable

Figure 7.3 Configurations of two-headed SPECT camera.

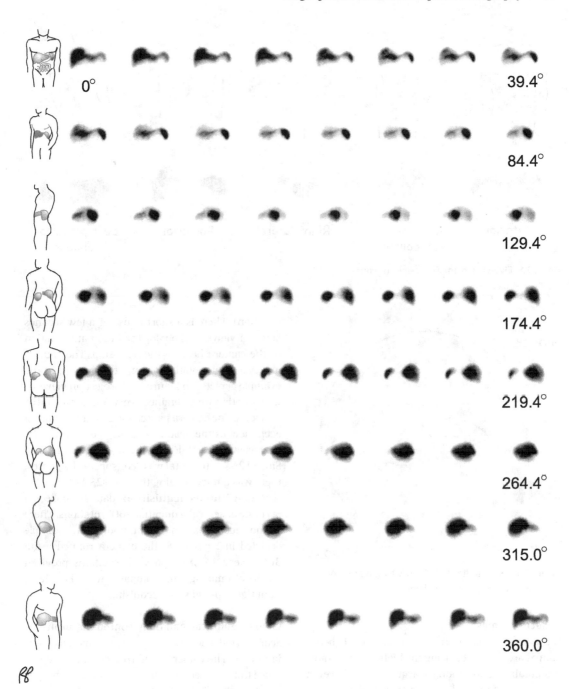

Figure 7.4 Projection views from a SPECT acquisition.

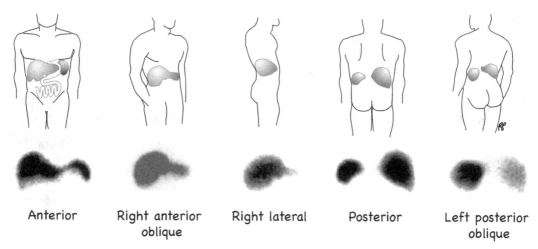

| Anterior | Right anterior oblique | Right lateral | Posterior | Left posterior oblique |

Figure 7.5 Five-view planar liver–spleen scan.

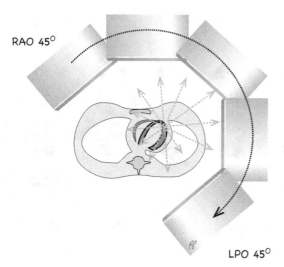

RAO 45°

LPO 45°

Figure 7.6 180° cardiac SPECT. (RAO, right anterior oblique; LPO, left posterior oblique.)

Collection times

For a given dose of radiopharmaceutical, better images are generated using the higher count statistics obtainable from longer acquisitions. However, patient comfort and cooperation limit imaging times. Acquisition times of 20–40 s per projection view are standard.

Step-and-Shoot vs. Continuous Acquisition

The standard method for the collection of tomographic projection views is called **step-and-shoot acquisition**. In this technique, each projection view is acquired in its entirety at each angular **stop**

(position). There is a short pause of a few seconds between views to allow for the automatic rotation of the camera head to the next stop. The camera makes a single rotation around the patient. In the example depicted in Figure 7.7, projection views of 20 s duration were obtained every 5.6° for a total of 64 views. The camera paused for 2 s after acquiring each view as the head moved into position for the next view. The total acquisition time was 1408 s. Since 126 s of this total was "consumed" by pauses, there was a total imaging time of 1282 s.

In **continuous acquisition**, data are collected over one or several sequential 360° rotations. There are no pauses; rotation is continuous. In the example depicted in Figure 7.8, the camera rotated a full 360° every 140.8 s. Ten such rotations provided 1408 s of imaging time (compared with the 1282 s from the step-and-shoot acquisition).

Circular, elliptical, and body-contouring orbits

Scans on older systems were acquired with a **circular orbit**. The camera head rotated at a fixed distance from the center of the body. Since the body is more nearly elliptical than circular in cross section, the camera did not come as close to the organ as possible over a significant portion of its rotation. Because image resolution is better if the camera is as close to an organ as possible, **elliptical** and, more recently, **body-contouring** orbits allow the camera heads to more closely follow the contour of the body and therefore remain closer to the organ being imaged (Figure 7.9). The body-contouring

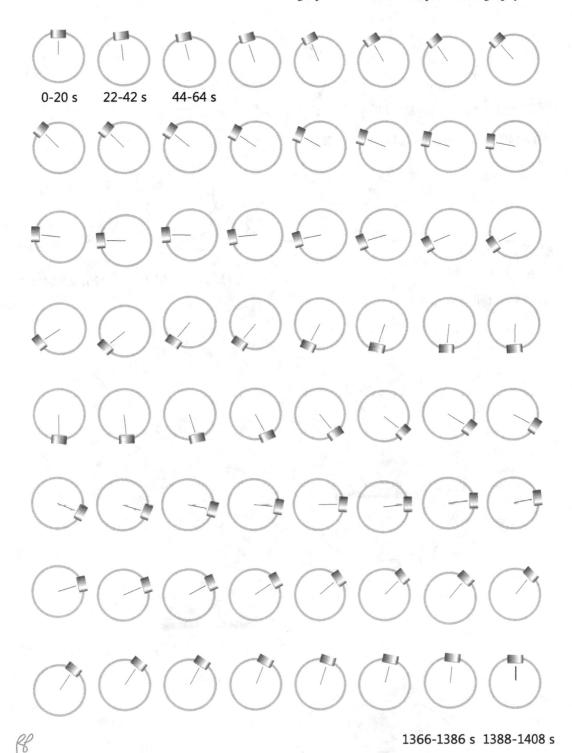

0-20 s   22-42 s   44-64 s

1366-1386 s   1388-1408 s

Figure 7.7 Step-and-shoot acquisition.

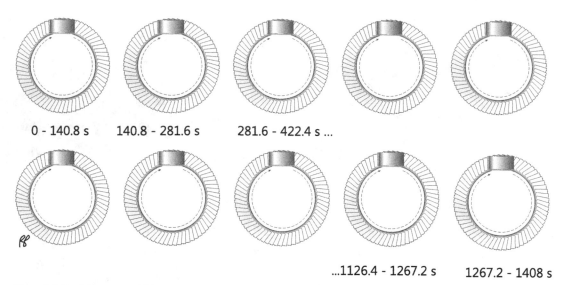

0 - 140.8 s   140.8 - 281.6 s   281.6 - 422.4 s ...

...1126.4 - 1267.2 s   1267.2 - 1408 s

Figure 7.8 Continuous acquisition.

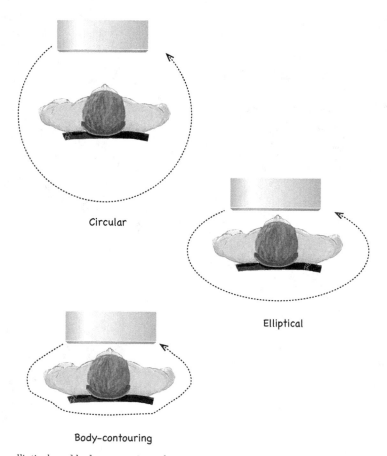

Circular

Elliptical

Body-contouring

Figure 7.9 Circular, elliptical, and body-contouring orbits.

orbits are enabled by electronic sensors placed on the collimators. As the gantry rotates, the detector radii are dynamically adjusted to get close to the body while avoiding collisions.

Patient motion and sinograms

Significant patient motion can cause artifacts or blurring in an image. To detect patient motion, the cine display and/or the sinogram (see below) should be reviewed prior to releasing the patient. Small amounts of patient motion can be corrected by automated correction algorithms that shift the projection views to align the organ of interest. Repeat acquisition is recommended if these algorithms are not successful.

A **sinogram** image is a stack of slices of the acquired projection views from 0° to the maximum angle of rotation, either 180° or 360°. Each row of the sinogram image consists of data acquired at a different angle of rotation, but all of the rows in the sinogram come from the same axial (y) position. In other words, there is a separate sinogram image for each slice location along the y-axis (the long axis) of the patient. Figure 7.10(a) is an illustration of the construction of a sinogram, representing a thin slice of the heart obtained from sample projection views from a 180° arc around the patient, and Figure 7.10(b) shows the complete sinogram, containing all of the projection views. Figure 7.11 shows sinograms taken at the level of the heart, the gallbladder, and the bowel. Figure 7.12 shows discontinuities seen in a sinogram of a patient who moved in the direction of the x-axis (side-to-side motion) and the y-axis (motion along the long axis) of his body during the acquisition of his images. It is not always possible to distinguish the direction of

motion from examination of the sinogram, but the cine images provide this information. Figure 7.13 is an example demonstrating artifacts created by patient motion in the direction of the y-axis. Correcting motion in the direction of the x-axis (created by side-to-side rotation or shifting in the axial plane) is more difficult than correcting motion in the direction of the y-axis (the long axis of the patient).

Dedicated cardiac SPECT cameras

A camera designed specifically for imaging the heart, as opposed to any organ or the whole body, can have a sensitivity advantage by focusing relatively large detectors at the relatively small space in the body containing the heart. In addition, since the application is limited, designers can simplify or optimize the gantry arrangement to reduce costs and improve patient comfort. Conventionally, cardiac imaging is performed on a general purpose two-headed SPECT camera with the heads oriented at (or close to) 90°; the gantry rotates approximately 90° to acquire the 180° of cardiac SPECT data (shown in Figure 7.6).

Dedicated cardiac cameras employ a similar strategy to sample photons over a limited arc with the patient upright, semireclined, or supine. Some of these camera designs are relatively minor variations on the general-purpose camera where multiple heads move to fill an arc of just over 180° (Figure 7.14(a)). Others employ apparently stationary heads but have moving internal detector assemblies (Figure 7.14(b)), and others employ completely stationary heads that sample the photons via multiple pinhole collimators (Figure 7.14(c)).

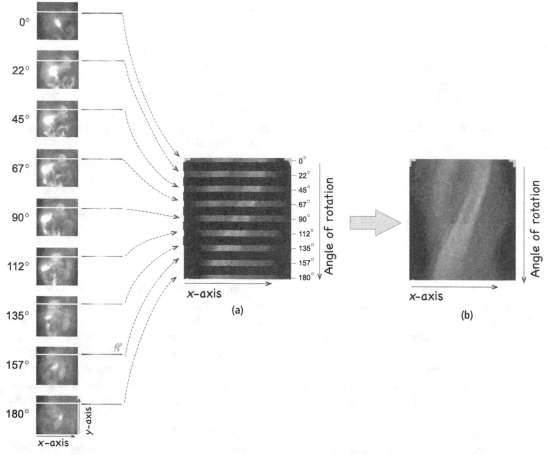

Figure 7.10 (a) Slices through the level of the heart from selected projection views are stacked to create a sinogram. (b) Complete sinogram.

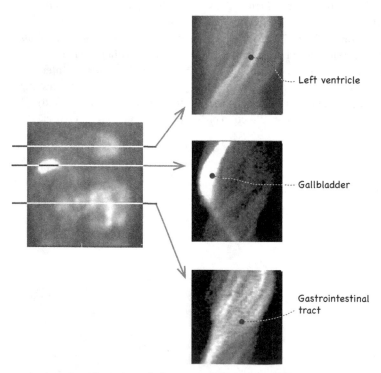

Figure 7.11 Sinograms at selected positions along the long axis of the body (*y*-axis).

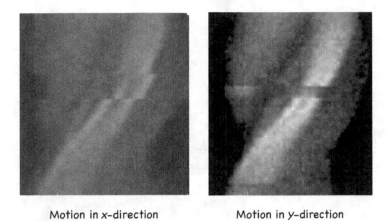

Motion in *x*-direction   Motion in *y*-direction

Figure 7.12 Effects of patient motion on sinograms of a slice of the heart.

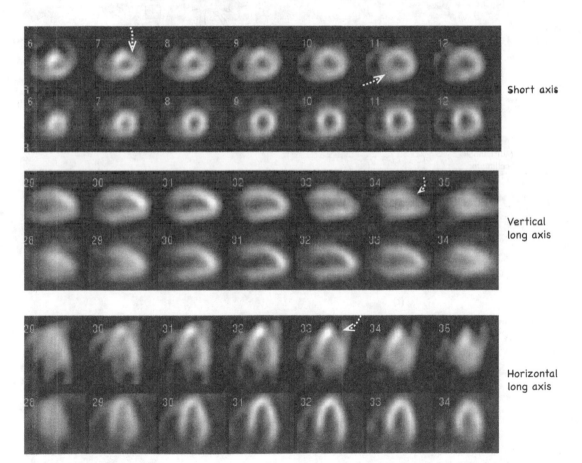

Short axis

Vertical
long axis

Horizontal
long axis

Figure 7.13 First, third, and fifth rows: artifacts created by patient motion (arrows). Second, fourth, and sixth rows: motion-corrected images.

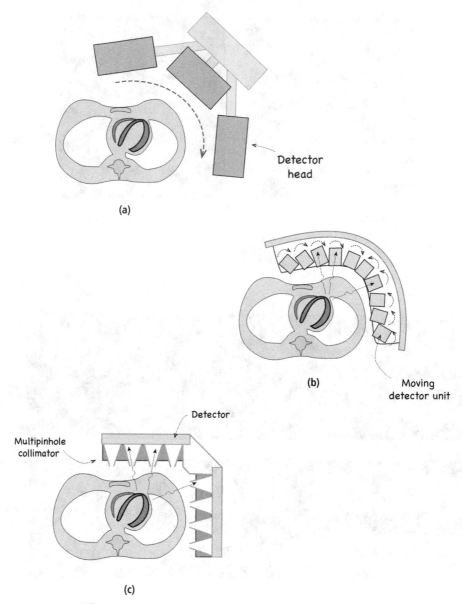

Figure 7.14 Newer cardiac SPECT cameras. (a) Multiple heads. (b) Stationary head with internal moving detector units. (c) Stationary head with pinhole collimators.

Questions

1. Match the following phrases to the terms listed below:
    (1) Individual images acquired at each stop of the SPECT camera as it rotates around the patient.
    (2) "Movie" of all of the projection views.
    (3) Reconstructed horizontal slices of the patient data.
    (4) A stack of slices from each acquired projection view, each slice taken at the same level of the body.

    Terms:
    (a) Cine views.
    (b) Projection views.
    (c) Sinogram.
    (d) Transverse slices.

2. True or false: Elliptical and body-contouring orbits for SPECT image acquisition improve image resolution compared with circular orbits because the camera remains closer to the patient as the heads rotate around the patient.

3. True or false: Examination of cine or sinogram images prior to discharging the patient from the nuclear medicine lab is no longer necessary, since motion correction software can compensate for almost any patient motion.

4. True or false: A 360° arc of acquisition is usually used for acquiring SPECT images of the heart, and a 180° arc is used for images of most other organs.

Answers

1. (1) (b). (2) (a). (3) (d). (4) (c).
2. True.
3. False: Software algorithms can only correct a small amount of motion.
4. False: The heart is eccentrically located in the chest, and therefore a 180° arc of rotation from the right anterior oblique projection to the left posterior oblique projection is used for cardiac SPECT imaging.

CHAPTER 8

Positron Emission Tomography

Positron emission tomography (PET) cameras are designed to detect the paired 511 keV photons generated from the annihilation event of a positron and electron. Following emission, any positron travels only a short distance before colliding with electrons in surrounding matter. As discussed in Chapter 2, the paired 511 keV annihilation photons travel in opposite directions (180° apart) along a line (Figure 8.1).

Following the acquisition of images of positron emissions, the data are reconstructed in a manner similar to that used for SPECT, with the exception that attenuation correction is always performed using a radionuclide transmission scan or, more commonly, CT data. PET has a number of advantages compared with SPECT. The most important are its greater sensitivity and resolution and the existence of positron-emitting isotopes of elements of low atomic number for which no suitable gamma emitters are available. The principal disadvantage of PET is the added cost of the equipment and the short half-life of some of the most useful positron emitters.

Advantages of PET imaging

Sensitivity

As pointed out earlier, a collimator reduces a camera's sensitivity because the collimator's septa cover part of the camera crystal's face. A collimator is not required for PET, since PET cameras use the detection of the simultaneous and oppositely directed 511 keV photons from positron annihilation to locate the direction from which the photons

originated. This is referred to as **annihilation coincidence detection**. In SPECT, the origins of the single photons can be located only if the camera is equipped with a collimator to absorb any photons not traveling perpendicular to the face of the crystal. Therefore a PET camera, needing no collimator, is inherently more sensitive (by at least a factor of 100) than a SPECT camera and has a higher count rate for similar quantities of radioactivity.

Resolution

Coincidence detection

If two detectors located on opposite sides of the annihilation reaction register coincident photon impacts, the annihilation reaction itself occurred along an imaginary line, called a **line of response** (LOR), drawn between these detectors (Figure 8.2). A **coincidence circuit** registers these as simultaneous events.

Events that arise from a single positron annihilation following the emission of a positron are referred to as **true coincidence events**. The impact of an unpaired photon, called a **singles event**, is rejected. A singles event is registered when an unpaired photon from a nonannihilation gamma ray impacts a detector (A in Figure 8.3). A singles event is also registered when only one of a pair of annihilation photons impacts a detector; the other photon may leave the plane of detection (B in Figure 8.3) or be absorbed or scattered by the surrounding medium (C in Figure 8.3).

Unfortunately, by chance, photons generated simultaneously from separate sites in the body may

Essentials of Nuclear Medicine Physics and Instrumentation, Third Edition. Rachel A. Powsner, Matthew R. Palmer, and Edward R. Powsner.
© 2013 John Wiley & Sons, Ltd. Published 2013 by John Wiley & Sons, Ltd.

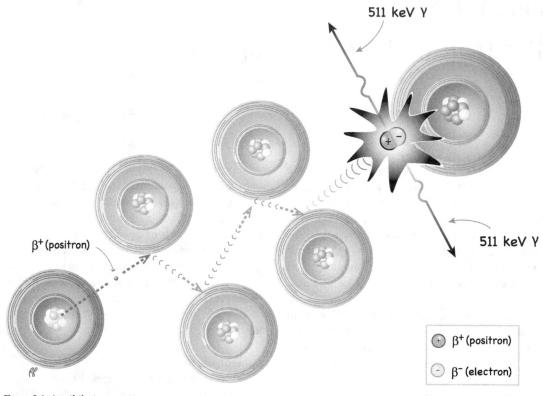

Figure 8.1 Annihilation reaction.

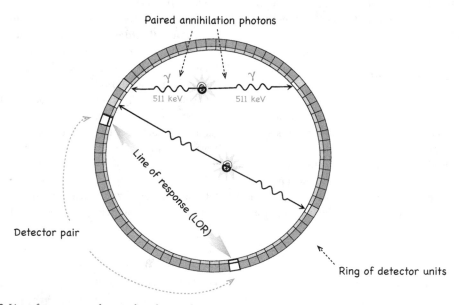

Figure 8.2 Line of response and examples of coincidence events.

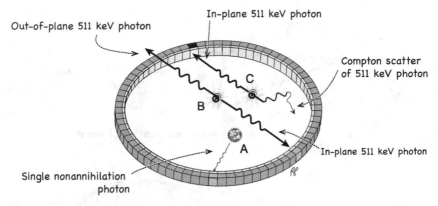

Out-of-plane 511 keV photon

In-plane 511 keV photon

Compton scatter of 511 keV photon

C

B

A

In-plane 511 keV photon

Single nonannihilation photon

Figure 8.3 Singles events.

reach the crystal at the same time. These separate events are incorrectly perceived as though resulting from annihilation of a single positron emission occurring along a line between the two detectors. These photons may arise from annihilation events (Figure 8.4(a)) when one photon from each member of a pair of annihilation events registers as a simultaneous event (their respective partners are out-of-plane events), or from simultaneous detection of nonannihilation photons (Figure 8.4(b)). Other mistakes in identification may also occur. For example, when scattering of one of the 511 keV photons alters its path, the location of the annihilation event may incorrectly be presumed to be on a line connecting the detectors (Figure 8.4(c)). These events are referred to as **random events** (a sort of false positive). The probability of random events increases significantly with increasing radioactivity within the field of view of the scanner, and such events are of most concern at high count rates. Scatter and random events are undesirable because they contribute to an increase in image background counts and consequently cause a reduction in image contrast.

Time of flight

To improve resolution, some systems also measure **time of flight** under the assumption that the annihilation can be localized along the line of flight of the coincident photons by measuring the time of arrival of each of the photons at the opposing crystals. Unless the event occurs in the exact center of the detection ring, one of the photons will arrive before the other. The time difference will be proportional to the difference in distances traveled by the

two photons and can be used to calculate the position of the event along the line connecting the detectors (Figure 8.5). Unfortunately, owing to current electronic-timing limitations, the calculated position of the annihilation event is not precise (Figure 8.6). However, knowing the approximate location of the annihilation event helps constrain the reconstruction algorithm and does provide information that is used to improve the quality of the image.

Radiopharmaceuticals

One of the greatest advantages of PET imaging is the large number of low-atomic-number elements for which positron emitters exist (Table 8.1). This permits incorporation of positron emitters into many biologically active compounds, including isotopic forms of oxygen, carbon, nitrogen, and fluorine. Very specific physiologic properties of an organ can therefore be imaged; for example, the oxygen consumption and the glucose metabolism of the brain can be independently imaged using $[^{15}O]_2$ and ^{18}F-fluorodeoxyglucose. Other radiopharmaceuticals that can be used in PET are listed in Table 8.2.

PET camera components

A PET detector commonly consists of rings of crystals (Figure 8.7). The rings may or may not be separated by septa. Each individual detector contains one or more large, segmented crystals or a collection of small crystals. A standard **detector unit**, or **block**, consists of a group of small crystals watched by photomultiplier tubes (PMTs); one such arrangement consists of 36 small crystals arranged in a 6×6 matrix, coupled to four PMTs.

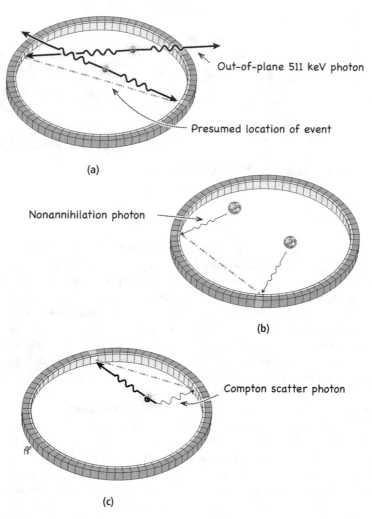

Figure 8.4 Random events.

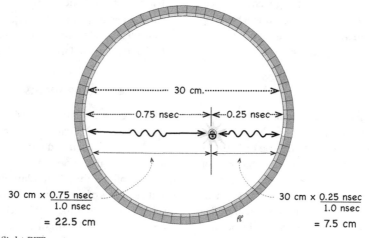

Figure 8.5 Time-of-flight PET systems.

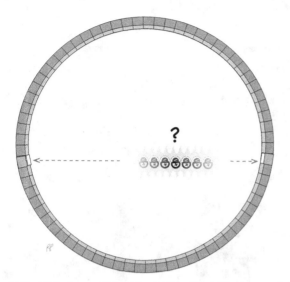

Figure 8.6 Current limitation of time-of-flight technology.

Table 8.1 Common positron-emitting nuclides. Data from [4]

Nuclide	Half-life (min)	Positron yield (%)	Maximum energy (MeV)	Method of production
^{11}C	20.3	99.8	0.960	Cyclotron
^{13}N	9.96	99.8	1.198	Cyclotron
^{18}F	109.77	96.7	0.633	Cyclotron
^{15}O	2.04	99.9	1.732	Cyclotron
^{82}Rb	1.26	95.5	3.378	Generator
^{68}Ga	67.71	88.9	1.899	Generator

Table 8.2 Examples of PET radiopharmaceuticals

Radiopharmaceutical	Physiologic imaging application
$[^{15}O]_2$	Cerebral oxygen metabolism and extraction
$H_2[^{15}O]$	Cerebral and myocardial blood flow
$C[^{15}O]$	Cerebral and myocardial blood volume
$[^{11}C]$-methionine	Tumor localization
$[^{11}C]$-choline	Tumor localization
$[^{18}F]$-fluorodeoxyglucose	Cerebral and myocardial glucose metabolism and tumor localization
$[^{13}N]H_3$	Myocardial blood flow
$[^{11}C]$-acetate	Myocardial metabolism
$[^{82}Rb]$	Myocardial blood flow

Crystals

The basic function of the crystal, of converting gamma photon energy into light photon energy, was discussed in Chapter 5. Thallium-doped sodium iodide (NaI(Tl)) crystals were originally used for PET systems; however, NaI has a relatively low density and is less effective at stopping the high-energy 511 keV photons. To compensate for the lower density, thicker crystals were employed for 511 keV imaging than those used for detecting the lower-energy single-photon emissions (3.8 cm as opposed to 0.6–1.2 cm).

Crystals with higher densities and higher atomic numbers (Z), such as bismuth germanate oxide (BGO), lutetium orthosilicate (LSO), and gadolinium orthosilicate (GSO), have been developed for use with 511 keV imaging owing to their greater stopping power for annihilation photons. This is because the likelihood of a photon interaction per unit volume increases linearly with density, and the probability of photoelectric interactions increases rapidly with increasing Z (it is proportional to Z^3) (see Figure 2.1 in Chapter 2). In detector design, photoelectric interactions are favored over Compton interactions since most of the energy from the photon is transmitted to the photoelectron, and the electron, being a charged particle, will deposit most of this energy in the material close to the location of the initial interaction (see Chapter 2). If, on the other hand, the initial interaction involving a 511 keV photon and the detector crystal is a Compton scatter event, only a small amount of the energy is transferred to an electron and deposited locally, and much of the energy of the scattered photon may escape the crystal.

LSO and GSO have the advantage of a shorter **decay time** than BGO or NaI(Tl) for PET imaging. The decay time is the time required for the radiation-excited atoms in the crystal lattice to return to the ground (unexcited) state with the emission of light photons (see Figure 5.2 and associated text). During this time, a second gamma photon entering the crystal cannot be detected. A shorter decay time is desirable for rapid imaging (see the section on dynamic images in Chapter 6).

A higher **light yield** is desirable because the greater the light photon output from the crystal per keV of absorbed gamma energy, the greater the energy resolution and the better the spatial resolution. Improved energy resolution improves

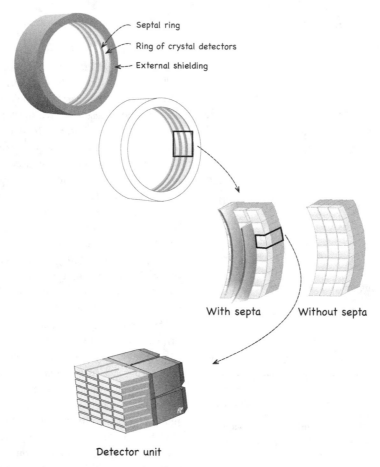

Septal ring
Ring of crystal detectors
External shielding

With septa / Without septa

Detector unit

Figure 8.7 PET camera.

the ability to distinguish the lower-energy scattered photons from the high-energy annihilation photons. The larger number of light photons makes it easier to identify which crystal has been struck by the annihilation photon, thereby improving spatial resolution. As outlined in Table 8.3, the choice of crystal material involves a compromise among the factors of cost, density, decay time, and light yield. Currently, LSO and a similar composite, LYSO (lutetium–yttrium orthosilicate), are the predominant crystals used in the manufacture of PET systems.

Photomultiplier tubes

The basic function of a PMT was discussed in Chapter 5 (see Figure 5.5). Unlike single-photon imaging systems, where many PMTs are attached to a single large crystal, positron cameras are designed with many crystal subdivisions watched by a few PMTs. The slits between crystal subdivisions channel the light photons toward the PMTs. Localization of the site of impact is achieved by measuring the light detected in each PMT; the closer the PMT is to the site of impact, the stronger the signal generated by the PMT (Figure 8.8).

Pulse-height analyzers, timing discriminators, and coincidence circuits

The signals from the PMTs are amplified by preamplifiers and amplifiers (see Figure 5.5 and associated text). The system electronics must then determine which signals came from paired 511 keV coincident photons arising from an annihilation event occurring along a line of response between a pair of

Table 8.3 Properties of crystals used for PET imaging

Crystal	Density (g/cm³)	Decay time (ns)	Light yield relative to NaI (%)
NaI(Tl)[a] (sodium iodide)	3.67	230	100
GSO (gadolinium orthosilicate)	6.71	060	041
BGO (bismuth germanate oxide)	7.13	300	014
LSO (lutetium orthosilicate)	7.40	040	075

Data from 5.6

[a] 3.8 cm thick (compared with 0.6–1.2 cm thick for single-photon emission cameras).

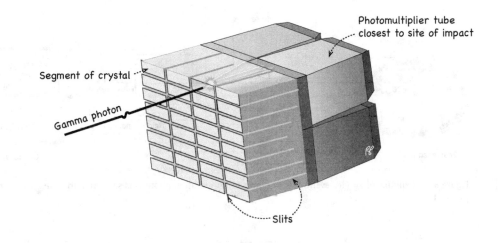

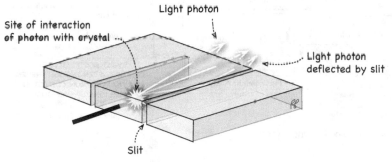

Figure 8.8 Slits between crystals direct light photons toward PMTs.

opposing detectors. This is accomplished primarily by measuring the size of each signal, which is proportional to the energy of the photon reaching the crystal, and by recording the time of detection of the signal. The pulse-height analyzer (Figure 5.6) determines whether the signal has the correct amplitude (pulse height) to have come from a 511 keV photon interaction within the crystal. The **timing discriminator** records the time the signal was generated. The **coincidence circuit** then examines signals of adequate amplitude coming from opposing detectors and determines whether the timing of the signals occurred within the **coincidence time window**. Typically, this coincidence time window is set to 5–15 ns, depending on the decay time of the selected crystal material.

As illustrated in Figure 8.9, two 511 keV coincident photons coming from an annihilation event along the line of response between a pair of detectors will yield adequately sized pulses and a timing

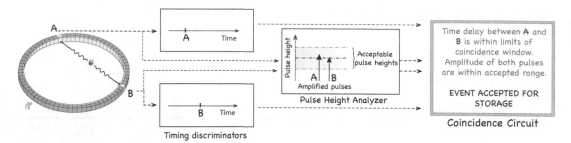

Figure 8.9 A coincidence event is accepted after processing by the pulse-height analyzers, timing discriminators, and coincidence circuits.

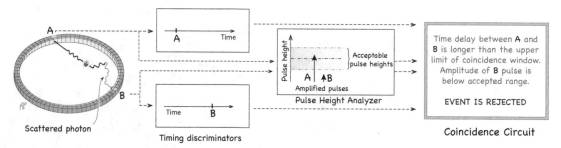

Figure 8.10 Example of singles event: one of a pair of annihilation photons is scattered and the corresponding data are rejected.

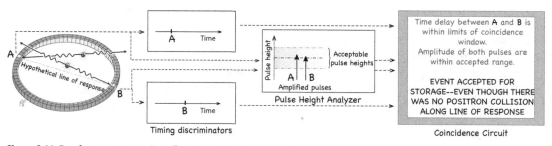

Figure 8.11 Random events can "pass" as true coincidence events.

delay that is less than the upper limit of the coincidence window. A coincidence event between the detector pairs will be recorded by the computer. In contrast, paired annihilation photons in which one or both of the photons have been subjected to scatter or absorption by surrounding tissue will usually be discarded by the coincidence circuit, as seen in Figure 8.10. This is because scattered photons have lower energies and because, in the process of scattering, the photon is often delayed on its path to the crystal. Random events are more difficult to separate from coincidence events, since they occur as the result of two 511 keV (or other

high-energy) photons arising from events occurring away from the line of response, but reaching the opposing detectors within the coincidence time window (Figure 8.11). Some systems estimate random-event rates arithmetically using a product of the coincidence time window and measured singles rates. Other approaches are available, but are beyond the scope of this text.

Septa

Septal rings can be used to improve resolution by reducing the amount of scatter from photons originating outside the plane of one ring of crystals.

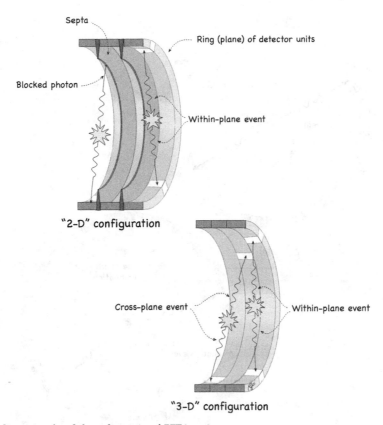

Figure 8.12 Two-dimensional and three-dimensional PET imaging.

The sensitivity of the scanner is reduced, however, because a significant fraction of true coincidence events are rejected. Removal of the septa will increase sensitivity and decrease resolution. Scans obtained with the septa in place are called **two-dimensional scans**; without septa, the scans are called **three-dimensional scans**. In the "2-D" illustration in Figure 8.12, the septa block out-of-plane photons, allowing only within-plane coincidence events to be recorded. The "3-D" configuration permits coincident registration of cross-plane events, those in which the two 511 keV photons are detected in different rings. Septa reduce the number of random coincidence events.

Factors affecting resolution in PET imaging

Positron range in tissue

Positrons travel a short distance in tissue before undergoing annihilation with an electron. Therefore, the camera detects photons originating from an annihilation event at a distance from the true source of the beta particle emission (Figure 8.13(a)). For lower-energy beta emitters (such as ^{18}F), this range is fairly small (1.2 mm in water); for higher-energy beta emitters (such as ^{82}Rb), the distance traveled prior to detection can be quite large (12.4 mm in water) [1]. The minimum possible resolving power of any system for a positron nuclide is therefore limited to the average range of the positrons in the tissue.

Photon emissions occurring at other Than 180°

Another factor causing degradation in resolution is the fact that 511 keV annihilation photons do not always travel in paths separated by exactly 180°. This is because the positron–electron combination will often be in motion during the process of annihilation, thereby altering the angle of ejection of the 511 keV photons. The detectors, however, assume a standard 180° emission path of the photons and therefore the localization of the positron emission is miscalculated in these cases (Figure 8.13(b)).

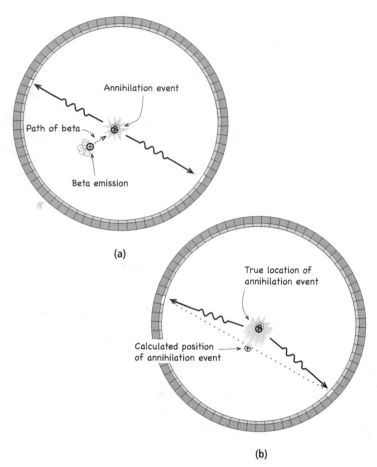

Figure 8.13 Factors limiting resolution in PET imaging.

Parallax error

Resolution decreases toward the periphery of a ring of PET detectors. This is because some of the photons arising from peripheral annihilation events cross the ring of detectors at an oblique angle and can interact with one of several detectors along a relatively long path. When a photon interacts within a detector, it is assumed the annihilation event occurred along a line of response originating at the front of the detector, since the depth of interaction in the crystal is not recorded. The illustrations in Figure 8.14(a) and (b) show two different possible lines of response (involving two different pairs of detectors) for a single annihilation event occurring near the edge of the ring of detectors. This effect is sometimes referred to as a **parallax error** or **depth-of-interaction effect**.

The larger the size of the ring of detectors, relative to the size of the body being imaged, the less

the effect, since the annihilation events will be more centrally located and the photons will cross the detector at a less oblique angle. This is illustrated in Figure 8.14(c), where the opposing photons from an annihilation event each cross two detectors in the smaller ring, and only one in the larger ring.

Attenuation in PET imaging

Because of the relatively high energy of the positron annihilation photons and the use of coincidence detection, attenuation correction is simpler and more accurate in PET than it is in SPECT. The attenuation coefficient for 511 keV photons as used in PET is more nearly uniform across the various kinds of body tissues (e.g., fat, muscle, and bone) than it is for the lower-energy photons encountered in SPECT. Also, the sum of the

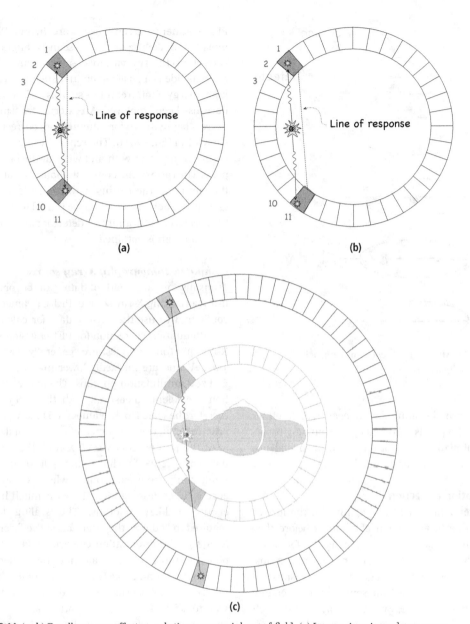

Figure 8.14 (a, b) Parallax error affects resolution near periphery of field. (c) Larger ring size reduces error.

likelihoods of absorption of the two photons of the 511 keV pair will be the same regardless of the location of the annihilation event along the line of response. Figure 8.15 illustrates the paths of paired annihilation photons originating at different positions along the line. For example, for every position along this line of response, the length of the path traversed by the photon traveling to the right increases the farther the annihilation has occurred

from the point at which the photon exits. This increase is exactly offset by the decrease in the length of the path traversed by the left-traveling photon of the pair. In other words, by adding the length of the path to the right to that for its pair-mate traveling to the left, one can see that the total amount of tissue traversed and therefore the total likelihood of absorption for the two photons of a pair will be the same no matter where along the line

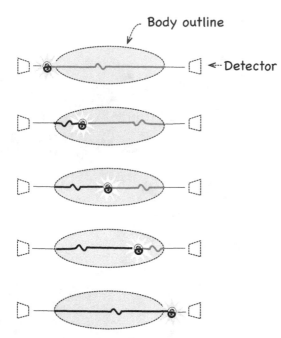

Figure 8.15 Attenuation is constant along a line connecting two detectors.

of response the annihilation occurred. If either photon of a pair is absorbed by surrounding tissue, the annihilation will not register as a coincidence event, and will not be counted.

Attenuation correction

The attenuation in PET imaging, i.e., the loss of counts due to absorption of photons before they arrive at the detector, is compensated for arithmetically by using data from transmission scans. Depending on the camera design, the transmission source can be a positron source, a high-energy single-photon source, or a CT X-ray source. Each approach has unique advantages and disadvantages. In any case, the number of counts in each line of response with the patient in place is compared with that without the patient in place to determine how much the count must be increased to compensate for the effect of absorption of photons in the patient's body.

External transmission source

This attenuation correction method uses a line source containing a long-lived radionuclide that orbits the space between the patient and the detectors. This somewhat outmoded scheme (almost all

PET scanners currently sold are hybrid PET-CT units and make use of the CT scan for attenuation correction) has two variants—most commonly, the radionuclide is a positron emitter such as ^{68}Ge, but high-energy photon emitters such as ^{137}Cs (662 keV) have also been employed. An external transmission source being used for attenuation correction is shown in Figure 8.16. The scheme works by comparing count rates with and without the patient in place. The ratio of the counts without the patient in the gantry to the counts with the patient in the gantry for each line of response is used to calculate the correction factor for this detector pair when the emission scan is obtained.

Computed-tomography X-ray source

Transmission attenuation data can be obtained using a rotating X-ray source. PET-CT cameras are configured to use their X-ray data for calculating the attenuation correction for PET emission scans. X-ray photon energies are generally less than 140 keV, and are markedly lower than that of the 511 keV annihilation photons. The linear attenuation coefficients measured with the X-rays must therefore be scaled to the values for 511 keV photons prior to being used to correct the emission data.

At the photon energies of X-rays, the attenuation coefficients for bone and soft tissue differ significantly from each other, whereas the difference is much less significant for the much higher-energy 511 keV photons. The scaling factors required to "adjust" the attenuation coefficients for X-rays to the attenuation coefficients for 511 keV photons must compensate for the differences between bone and soft tissue. To accomplish this, more than one scale factor is used to convert the CT scan to a 511 keV-equivalent attenuation map. To enact that transformation, the usual logic is to assume that values with CT numbers less than that of water (HU = 0) represent a mix of air and soft tissue, values greater than that of water represent a mix of bone and soft tissue, and values greater than some threshold represent pure bone (Figure 8.17).

Following the calculation of the 511 keV-equivalent attenuation map, projections are computed for each of the detector lines of response to obtain the total attenuation expected along each ray, and these values are used for attenuation correction of the PET projections.

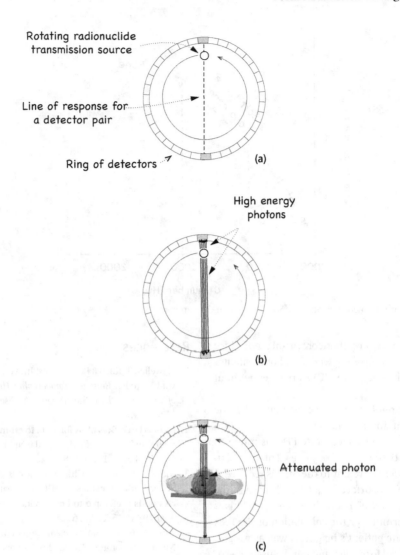

Rotating radionuclide
transmission source

Line of response for
a detector pair

Ring of detectors   (a)

High energy
photons

(b)

Attenuated photon

(c)

Figure 8.16 Radionuclide transmission source for PET attenuation correction. (a) Rotating high-energy transmission source (positron or single-photon) and sample line of response. (b) Transmission scan without patient. (c) Transmission scan with patient in place.

Standard uptake values

Determination of the amount of an injected radionuclide that is taken up by a tumor or organ is used in ^{18}F-fluorodeoxyglucose (FDG) scans to aid in the differentiation of benign from malignant masses and to follow tumor progression and/or posttreatment regression. Because accurate measurement of uptake is confounded by, among other things, the variable and often poorly known extent of photon absorption in the surrounding tissues, a semiquantitative measure, the **standard uptake value**

(SUV), is commonly used as an estimate of the actual uptake.

Calculation of the SUV requires a PET estimate of the concentration of activity in the tumor or organ in millicuries per milliliter or millibecquerels per milliliter, the mass of the patient in grams, and the amount of the injected activity in millicuries or millibecquerels:

$$\text{SUV} = (\text{concentration of activity in the tumor in mBq/ml}) \times (\text{mass of the patient in g})/(\text{injected activity in mBq})$$

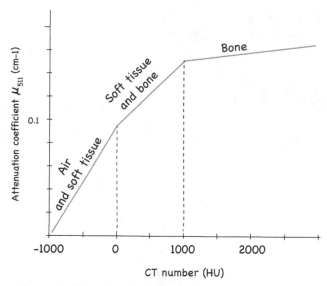

Figure 8.17 Attenuation coefficients for ^{18}F PET based on CT numbers.

The units of SUV are therefore g/mL, but since tissue is almost completely water, and one milliliter of water weighs one gram, SUVs are given without units.

SUV measurements are overestimated by the above formula in patients who are overweight, because fat does not concentrate FDG as much as the rest of the tissue of the body does. The contribution of the patient's weight to the SUV is reduced if the patient's body surface area (BSA) is used in the calculation instead of his or her mass [3]. This is because the formula for the calculation of the BSA incorporates the patient's height as well as weight. There are several formulas that can be used to estimate BSA; one example is [2]

$$\text{Body surface area} = (\text{weight in kg})^{0.425}$$
$$\times (\text{height in cm})^{0.725} \times 0.007184$$

The formula for SUV based on body surface area becomes

$$SUV_{BSA} = (\text{concentration of activity in the tumor interest}) \times (\text{body surface area})/(\text{injected activity})$$

References

1. Llewellen T, Karp J. Pet systems. In: Wernick MN, Aarsvold JN (eds.) *Emission Tomography: The Fundamentals of PET and SPECT*. San Diego, CA: Elsevier, 2004, pp. 179–194.
2. DuBois D, DuBois EF. A formula to estimate the approximate surface area if height and weight be known. *Arch Int Med* 1916; 17:863–871.
3. Kim CK, Gupta NC, Chandramouli B, Alavi A. Standardized uptake values of FDG: body surface area correction is preferable to body weight correction. *J Nucl Med* 1994; 35:164–167.
4. NuDat 2.6, National Nuclear Data Center, Brookhaven National Laboratory, NuDat 2.6, January 12, 2012. http://www.nndc.bnl.gov/nudat2/chartNuc.jsp. (accessed 10 December 2012)
5. Early PJ. Positron emission tomography (PET). In: Early PJ, Sodee DB (eds.) *Principles and Practice of Nuclear Medicine*. St. Louis: CV Mosby, 1995, p. 319.
6. Ficke DC, Hood JT, TerPogossian MM. A spheroid positron emission tomograph for brain imaging: A feasibility study. *J Nucl Med* 1996; 37:1219–1225.

Questions

1. Match the following phrases with the choices listed below the phrases:
   (a) Two 511 keV photons arising from a single annihilation event striking opposing detectors simultaneously.
   (b) Two 511 keV photons arising from separate annihilation events striking opposing detectors simultaneously.
   (c) One 511 keV photon from a single annihilation event strikes a detector, and the other is absorbed by surrounding tissue.

   Choices: singles event, random event, true coincidence event.

2. Which of the following characteristics are desirable for the crystalline materials used to detect 511 keV photons?
   (a) Low density.
   (b) High atomic number.
   (c) Long decay time.
   (d High light yield.

3. True or false: Coincidence circuitry can more readily differentiate singles events from true coincidence events than random events from true coincidence events.

4. Which of the following factors tend to reduce resolution in PET imaging?
   (a) The positrons can travel a significant distance prior to annihilation.
   (b) Septa in 3-D imaging decrease the number of detected true coincidence events.
   (c) 511 keV photon emissions are not always exactly 180° apart following an annihilation reaction.
   (d) Proximity of the source to the edge of the ring of detectors.

5. Which of the following are true about current "time of flight" annihilation detection technology on PET scanners?
   (a) Precise localization of the position of an annihilation event along a line of response is possible.
   (b) Approximate localization of an annihilation event along a line of response can be used to improve image quality.

6. True or false: Standard uptake value (SUV) measurements based on body surface area may be more accurate than those based on weight alone in obese patients because adipose tissue does not concentrate FDG as much as the rest of the tissue in the body.

Answers

1. (a) True coincidence event. (b) Random event.
   (c) Singles event.
2. (b) and (d). High density and short decay are preferable; (a) and (c) are incorrect.
3. True.
4. (a), (c), and (d). (b) is incorrect because septa have nothing to do with 3-D scanning.
5. (b).
6. True.

CHAPTER 9

X-ray Computed Tomography

Computed tomography (CT) is a three-dimensional imaging modality based on X-ray imaging. In a CT scanner, multiple planar X-ray images are acquired and then processed mathematically to create cross-sectional images through the body. Relative to nuclear imaging, CT scanners are capable of low-noise, high-resolution, detailed anatomical images and are therefore highly complementary. As a result, the hybrid imaging techniques of PET-CT and SPECT-CT have now emerged in the nuclear medicine clinic, and so an understanding of X-rays and CT scanners is essential for the nuclear medicine professional.

In this chapter, we shall briefly introduce X-ray tubes and how they produce X-rays. We shall then discuss the general configuration of a CT scanner.

X-ray production

Wilhelm Roentgen is usually credited with discovering X-rays. Although they had been observed earlier, Roentgen was the first to describe their basic properties, in 1895, and in 1901, he was awarded the first Nobel Prize in Physics. When he first observed them, the nature of the radiation was unknown and its properties surprising, if not actually mysterious. This is reflected in his use of the "X" in naming them "X-rays."

A modern **X-ray tube** (Figure 9.1) is an evacuated glass or ceramic tube with a window for the exiting X-rays. Within the vacuum tube, electrons are "boiled off" an electrically heated filament wire, the **cathode**, and are accelerated to high speed toward a positively charged tungsten target, the **anode**, by a high potential difference (or voltage)

maintained between the filament and the target (Figure 9.2). The vast majority of these electrons interact with outer-shell electrons of the tungsten target and their kinetic energy is lost as heat. A small percentage of the electrons bombarding the target, approximately 0.2% of them, cause the emission of an X-ray by either characteristic radiation or bremsstrahlung (see Chapter 2).

Medical imaging utilizes both characteristic and bremsstrahlung X-rays. Although characteristic X-rays have discrete, or specific, energies, bremsstrahlung interactions produce a full range of X-ray energies, from 0 keV to a maximum that is equal to the **maximum** or **peak voltage** applied between the filament and target. The energy of each bremsstrahlung X-ray is dependent upon the proximity of the moving electron and the nucleus of a nearby atom involved in the bremsstrahlung interaction. The closer the electron comes to the nucleus, the greater the deceleration of the electron and the greater the energy of the X-ray produced by this interaction (for an illustration of bremsstrahlung, see Figure 2.13). The larger the peak applied voltage (expressed in kilovolts and abbreviated as **kVp**) between the filament and the target in the X-ray tube, the higher the maximum bremsstrahlung X-ray energy and the greater the number of X-rays created. An energy spectrum of a typical X-ray beam is shown by the dashed line in Figure 9.3.

The lowest-energy X-rays in the X-ray beam add to the radiation dose to the patient, particularly to the skin, but are not penetrating enough to reach the detectors and contribute to the image quality. The glass of the vacuum tube blocks some of the lowest-energy X-rays, and others are attenuated

Essentials of Nuclear Medicine Physics and Instrumentation, Third Edition. Rachel A. Powsner, Matthew R. Palmer, and Edward R. Powsner.

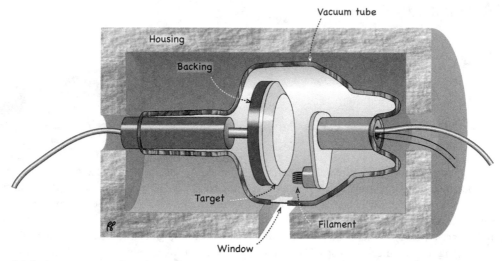

Figure 9.1 Basic components of an X-ray tube.

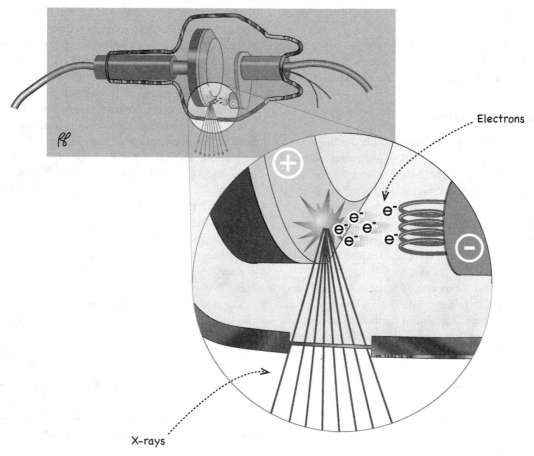

Figure 9.2 X-rays are generated when electrons strike the tungsten target.

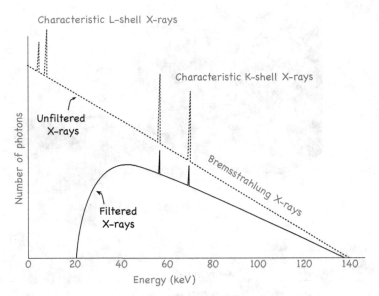

Figure 9.3 X-ray spectrum.

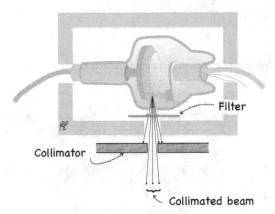

Figure 9.4 The filter attenuates the lower-energy X-rays (depicted as lighter gray arrows) and a collimator narrows the X-ray beam.

by a **filter** (usually aluminum) placed in front of the tube window (Figure 9.4). Thus both the applied voltage between the filament and target and the attenuation by the filter affect the range of energies of the X-rays delivered to the patient (solid line in Figure 9.3). In addition, the amount of electricity or current (expressed in milliamperes (mA)) used to heat the filament to boil off the electrons and the duration of this current (in seconds) affect the total number of X-rays emitted. The last two quantities

are often combined as a product and referred to as **mAs** (milliamperes-seconds). Finally, the X-ray beam is narrowed, or **collimated**, by lead shutters (Figure 9.4) to avoid irradiating tissues other than those being imaged.

In general, the greater the kVp and mAs the better the image quality, but the greater the radiation dose delivered to the patient. When one is setting the kVp and mAs parameters, particularly in CT imaging, a balance can be achieved between obtaining the image quality needed for clinical diagnosis and keeping the radiation dose to the patient as low as possible.

An unavoidable accompaniment of bombardment of the target is the generation of **heat**. The tungsten itself is dense enough to stop the electrons and capable of withstanding the heating. The heat is dissipated from the tungsten by a copper backing and by rapid rotation of the target, which spreads the heat over a larger area and allows a brief rest period for any one spot to "cool down" before serving again as the focus point of the electron beam. Further methods of cooling include limiting the duration of the bombardment, and external air or oil cooling.

The contents of the X-ray tube are in a vacuum so that there are no gas particles to impede the flow of the electrons.

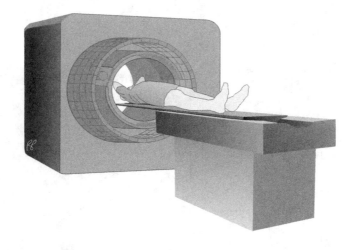

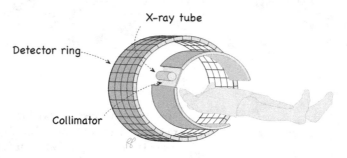

Figure 9.5 Basic components of one type of CT scanner, containing a stationary detector ring and rotating inner X-ray tube.

X-ray imaging

Images created by projecting X-rays at the body, also called "X-rays" by convention, are in essence shadows. They can be thought of as "inverse shadows": denser tissues such as bone, which block much of the X-rays, appear as white on a film or a digital detector, and lungs, which are composed mainly of air, appear to be very dark in the image.

Computed tomography

Overview

An X-ray of a patient taken using a stationary X-ray source and detector is called a planar image. Chest X-rays are probably the most common example of a planar X-ray image. If, on the other hand, the X-ray data is recorded over a full 360° path encircling the patient, this data can also be "back-projected" to create transaxial slices. The X-ray source and detectors in most current scanners are arranged in one of two configurations. Either the

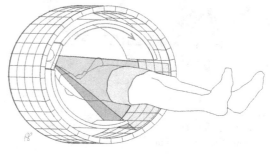

Figure 9.6 Rotate–stationary configuration. A rotating source and collimator generate a fan-shaped X-ray beam that is directed toward a stationary ring of detectors.

X-ray source rotates within a stationary complete ring of detectors (such systems are called **rotate–stationary** systems) as illustrated in Figures 9.5 and 9.6 or, more commonly, the X-ray source and an opposing arc of detectors rotate in synchrony around the patient (**rotate–rotate** systems) as seen in Figure 9.7. At the current time, rotate–stationary configurations are too expensive to manufacture for

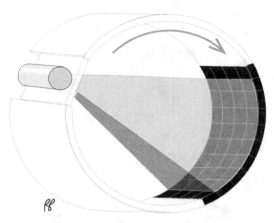

Figure 9.7 Rotate–rotate configuration. The opposing source and detector rotate synchronously.

multislice detectors (see below) and therefore rotate–rotate systems are the predominant configuration. The process of acquisition and reconstruction of X-ray data is called **computed (trans)axial tomography** (CAT) or simply **computed tomography** (CT) scanning.

The X-ray source is moved in increments around the patient. At each position, the X-ray tube is turned on and the patient is exposed to a fan-shaped beam of X-rays (Figures 9.6 and 9.7).

The X-rays that are not attenuated by the patient's body are registered by the detectors on the opposite side of the patient. The detectors are composed of **ceramic scintillators**, which, like the NaI(Tl) crystals discussed in Chapter 5, emit light in response to X-rays. Because the scintillator detectors used in CT scanners must respond to the large, rapidly changing flow of X-rays generated by the CT X-ray source, the chemical composition of the material in the ceramic is more complex than that of the NaI(Tl) crystal. In particular, these scintillators must have a very rapid decay time: both the initial light output in response to the X-ray excitation must be rapid and the residual light present within the scintillator after the initial response, called the **afterglow**, must dissipate rapidly.

The ceramic scintillators are backed by **photodiodes**, which generate electrical pulses or currents in response to the light photons. Photodiodes are semiconductor devices that function similarly to photomultiplier tubes (PMTs) by converting light photon energy into current. Semiconductors and PMTs are discussed in Chapters 4 and 5, respectively.

Multislice detector configurations

Older CT scanners were equipped with a single row of detectors. Most CT scanners are now manufactured with multiple detector rows arranged side by side along the z-axis of the scanner (Figure 9.8(a)) and are called multidetector or, more commonly, multislice CT scanners. Having multiple detector rows allows faster scanning times, as a larger area of the patient can be imaged during a single rotation of the X-ray tube. The total number of detector rows used during scanning is determined by the collimated width of the beam (Figure 9.8(b)).

Within each row, the detectors are of uniform size. On most new scanners, the innermost rows of detectors contain smaller detectors than the outermost rows. Single detector rows can be used to collect a "slice" of data or one or more adjacent rows of detectors can be "grouped" together and collected as a slice. The number of slices in a scanner's designation (such as "64-slice CT") refers to the number of simultaneous data slices, sometimes called data channels, that can be collected and not to the total number of detector rows. A four-slice or 16-slice scanner can have, for example, 16 or 32 detector rows. If the smallest detectors are each assigned to a slice or channel, then the images will have the finest detail or greatest resolution, but the scan acquisition time will be longer. If adjacent rows are grouped together, there will be a lower image resolution but the acquisition time will be faster. Figure 9.9 shows a hypothetical four-slice scanner with a detector array composed of 12 rows; the innermost eight rows are 0.5 mm wide and the outermost rows 1 mm wide. By grouping increasing numbers of detector rows (and widening the collimated beam), slices of width 0.5, 1, and 2 mm can be collected.

Axial and helical scanning

Older CT scanners acquired individual axial slices. The patient bed (pallet) was advanced in small increments. After each increment, the bed was stopped and an axial slice was acquired (Figure 9.10(a)). Newer CT scanners acquire continuously as the bed advances continuously, so that the path of the X-ray source is much like the peel of a tubular apple or a helix; therefore this is referred to as a **helical** scan (Figure 9.10(b)). Some authors use the name **spiral** instead of "helical" to refer to the same process.

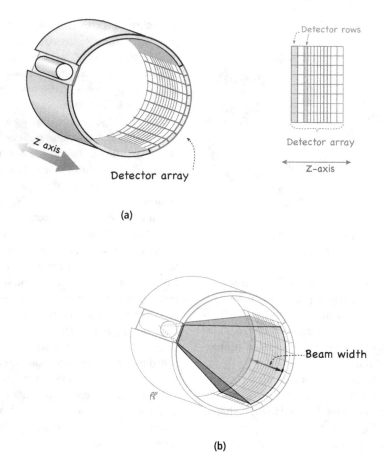

(a)

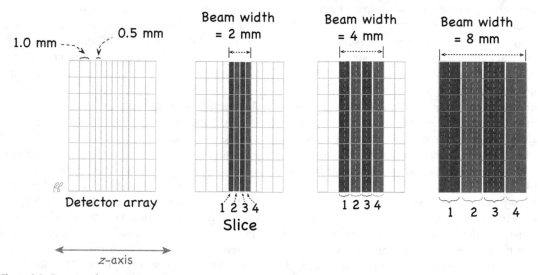

(b)

Figure 9.8 Multislice CT detector array composed of multiple rows of detectors placed side by side along the z-axis.

Figure 9.9 Grouping detector rows allows acquisition of slices of varying width.

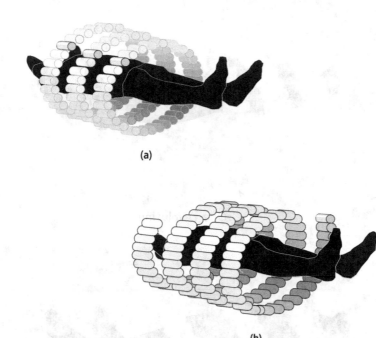

(a)

(b)

Figure 9.10 Axial versus helical scanning.

There are two advantages to helical scanning. The first is the shorter duration of the study owing to faster scanning times, and the second is the increased flexibility during data reconstruction. The angle of reconstruction of the axial slices can be chosen by the operator, and higher-quality coronal and sagittal slices can be created from the datasets.

Pitch

The helical motion of the gantry of the scanner can be described by specifying both the rotational speed of the gantry, in revolutions per second, and the distance the patient bed travels along the long axis of the patient, in millimeters for each revolution of the gantry. The latter is called the **pitch** of the helix, an engineering term for describing the threads of a screw or bolt. The uppermost illustration in Figure 9.11 shows an acquisition with a shorter distance traveled per revolution, or a smaller pitch, than in the lower illustration.

The pitch is defined mathematically as the distance the table travels divided by the summed widths of the detector rows being used for X-ray data collection, which is also the collimated X-ray beam width:

Pitch = table movement per rotation/

   beam width

Hounsfield units

CT pixel intensities are given in CT numbers or **Hounsfield units** (HU), and are simply scaled units of attenuation as measured by CT. The Hounsfield unit is named for Sir Godfrey Hounsfield, who developed the first practical CT scanner and who, along with Allan Cormack, was awarded the 1979 Nobel Prize in Medicine. It is not easily converted to SI units; nevertheless, radiology uses the Hounsfield unit for dose calculation in preference to the attenuation coefficient used by most other disciplines. If μ is the average linear attenuation coefficient for the pixel of interest and μ_w is the value for water, then the CT number in HU is given by

$$\text{HU} = (\mu - \mu_w)/\mu_w$$

Tables of attenuation values in Hounsfield units are available. Air, which stops virtually no X-radiation, has a value of $-1000\,\text{HU}$; water, which moderately attenuates the X-ray beam, has a value of $0\,\text{HU}$ (zero); and bone, which blocks a large fraction of the beam, has a value of $1000\,\text{HU}$ or greater. The HU value for fat is about -10, and the firmer of the soft body tissues have HU values in a range from about 10 to 60.

A more in-depth discussion of photon attenuation is given in Chapter 2.

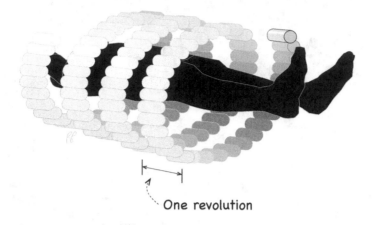

One revolution

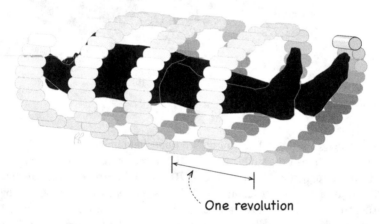

One revolution

Figure 9.11 Pitch.

Questions

1. True or false: X-ray production is an efficient process. The majority of electrons striking the tungsten target cause the emission of X-rays.

2. Which of the following statements are true about the X-ray beam produced by X-ray tubes?
   (a) The X-rays are monoenergetic: they all have the same energy in keV.
   (b) The beam is a combination of characteristic and bremsstrahlung radiation.
   (c) The maximum X-ray energy is not affected by the peak voltage applied between the filament and target.
   (d) The number of X-rays produced in the target increases as the current in the filament increases.

3. Which of the following statements are true concerning CT scanning?
   (a) CT images acquired in conjunction with PET images can provide useful correlative anatomic information.
   (b) Helical CT scanning allows faster acquisition times and greater flexibility in image reconstruction compared with conventional axial CT scanning.
   (c) Current CT scanners consist of a stationary ring of detectors with an inner rotating X-ray source or a rotating arc of detectors that oppose the rotating X-ray source.
   (d) All of the above.

4. True or false: A common definition of the term "pitch," when used in reference to helical CT scanning, is the ratio of the distance the patient bed advances per gantry revolution to the width of the collimated X-ray beam.

5. Select the numbers of Hounsfield units (HU) from the values below that most closely correspond to the following:
   (a) Bone.
   (b) Fat.
   (c) Muscle.
   (d) Air.
   (e) Water.

   HU values: $-1000, -10, 0, 30, 1000$.

6. What are the advantages of helical scanning?
   (a) Faster scan times.
   (b) Greater flexibility in angle of reconstruction of axial slices.
   (c) Higher-quality coronal and sagittal reconstruction views.
   (d) All of the above.

Answers

1. False: 98% of the kinetic energy of the electrons is lost as heat in the target.
2. (b) and (d) are correct.
3. (d).
4. True.
5. Bone, 1000. Fat, −10. Muscle, 30. Air, −1000. Water, 0.
6. (d).

CHAPTER 10

Hybrid Imaging Systems: PET-CT and SPECT-CT

For specific clinical diagnoses, positron emission tomography (PET) and single-photon computed tomography (SPECT) imaging can detect more sites of disease than can conventional anatomical imaging techniques such as X-ray computed tomography (CT) or magnetic resonance imaging (MRI). Interpretation of PET and SPECT images can be difficult, however, because these nuclear medicine images have few anatomical landmarks for determining the location of abnormal findings. Combining PET or SPECT with CT images acquired sequentially on separate devices provided a partial solution to this problem. Unless patient positioning was carefully reproduced between the studies, however, the nuclear medicine and X-ray images did not match, and the resulting misregistration led to inaccuracies in determining the anatomic location of the abnormalities seen in the nuclear medicine images. In one approach to correcting for positioning errors, the images from a PET or SPECT camera and a CT scanner were fused manually or by computer software or both. To further ensure accurate registration of the PET and CT data, the two imaging modalities have been physically combined in single units, the **PET-CT scanner** and the **SPECT-CT scanner**. These combined units also facilitate the use of the CT data to correct the nuclear medicine images for the attenuation of the gamma radiation as it traverses body tissues en route to the detectors.

PET-CT

PET-CT scanners are presently configured as sequential gantries, also called in-line cameras,

with a shared patient bed, or pallet. An illustration of a combined PET-CT scanner is shown in Figure 10.1. The advantage of this configuration, as discussed above, is the consistent positioning of the patient between the acquisitions, which reduces the risk of misregistration of the images. In addition, again as mentioned above, the CT data can be used for attenuation correction for the PET or SPECT images. Attenuation correction using CT data is discussed in Chapter 8.

In PET-CT configurations, the CT scanner is closer to the patient. The CT scan is normally acquired in its entirety prior to acquiring the PET scan (Figure 10.2), although the order of acquisition of the studies can be reversed.

SPECT-CT

All PET-CT scanners are currently manufactured with multislice CT units. Hybrid SPECT-CT scanners, however, are offered in a number of different configurations. In addition to the sequential gantry configuration, with the SPECT camera heads on a gantry closer to the patient, there are systems where both the SPECT camera heads and the CT X-ray tube and detectors are supported on a single rotating gantry (Figure 10.3). The latter solution is more compact (frequently requiring fewer room modifications for installation) and usually less expensive than the dual-gantry configurations. In addition, owing to their lower X-ray tube output, they require less room shielding.

There are some limitations of single-gantry systems, however. With both the X-ray tube and detectors and the SPECT heads mounted on a single

---

Essentials of Nuclear Medicine Physics and Instrumentation, Third Edition. Rachel A. Powsner, Matthew R. Palmer, and Edward R. Powsner.
© 2013 John Wiley & Sons, Ltd. Published 2013 by John Wiley & Sons, Ltd.

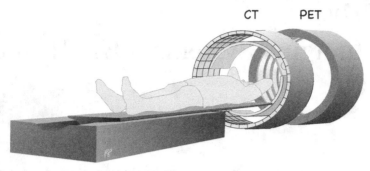

Figure 10.1 PET-CT.

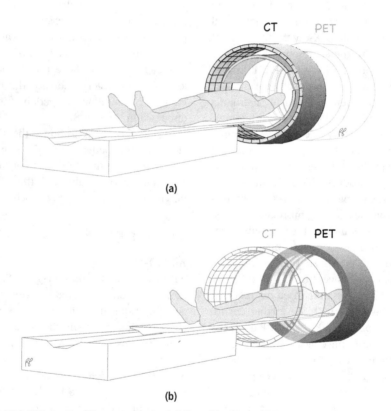

Figure 10.2 PET-CT. (a) The entire CT scan is acquired, followed by (b) the PET scan.

rotational system, the speed of rotation is limited and CT acquisition is slower than in systems with the CT scanner incorporated as a separate gantry. Consequently, artifacts from patient motion, both voluntary and involuntary, such as peristalsis of the gastrointestinal tract, are more common. As a result of patient motion and the lower X-ray tube output, the CT image quality is generally inferior to that from multislice systems.

Current limitations of hybrid imaging

Breathing artifacts

Hybrid cameras have mitigated the majority of the registration problems between the PET or SPECT and CT images caused by differences in patient positioning, which occur when the patient must be physically moved between independent systems (the nuclear medicine system and CT unit).

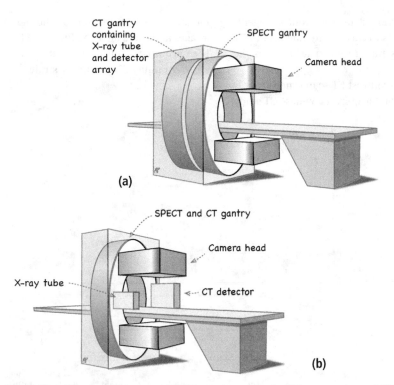

Figure 10.3 SPECT-CT. (a) Two-gantry system with CT system contained within one gantry and SPECT heads supported on a second gantry. (b) Single-gantry system with one gantry supporting both the SPECT camera heads and an X-ray tube and detector.

However, owing to differences in breathing patterns between CT imaging, where breath holding is desirable, and PET and SPECT imaging, where breath holding is not possible, misalignment, particularly near the diaphragm, can cause misregistration of images in the lower lungs and upper abdomen. In addition, if the CT data are used for attenuation correction, artifacts may be introduced into the PET or SPECT images in those areas. To ensure better alignment of the diaphragm, some institutions instruct patients to breathe normally or shallowly during both the CT and the PET or SPECT acquisition.

Contrast agent artifacts

The use of intravenous and oral contrast agents during CT imaging can improve anatomic localization; however, the contrast agent is relatively dense and can alter the attenuation maps that are constructed from the CT data. In particular, the X-ray attenuation will be greatly increased at sites of greater concentrations of contrast agent, such as sites of pooling of oral contrast in the colon or vascular filling with an intravenous bolus. Although the gamma photon emissions in both PET and SPECT imaging are also attenuated by contrast agents, the distribution of the contrast agent can change between the time of acquisition of the CT study and that of the PET or SPECT study. As a result, the CT attenuation map may not correctly approximate the gamma photon attenuation in the specific areas affected.

In addition, the HU value, or amount of X-ray attenuation, will also be somewhat increased in soft tissues into which the contrast agent diffuses. As a result, the scaling factors for the attenuation coefficients (see the section on attenuation correction in Chapter 8) of soft tissue, which are based on noncontrast CT X-ray attenuation, are not as accurate. For the above reasons, the use of attenuation correction data from contrast-agent-enhanced CT studies to correct attenuation in PET and SPECT studies may result in artifacts in the final images.

In cases where a contrast CT scan is needed, it is not uncommon to first acquire a low-dose CT study for attenuation correction of the gamma photon images and then, after the PET or SPECT study has been acquired, to inject contrast media and acquire a better-quality diagnostic CT study.

Questions

1. Artifacts in hybrid imaging can occur as the result of which of the following?
   (a) Breath holding following deep inspiration during CT acquisition followed by normal breathing during PET or SPECT acquisition.
   (b) Attenuation correction of PET or SPECT images with contrast CT images.
   (c) (a) and (b).

2. What are some of the advantages of using a hybrid imaging system?
   (a) Misregistration as a result of patient motion is reduced, as the patient remains on the same imaging pallet (bed) during acquisition of both the CT and the PET or SPECT images.
   (b) The CT images can be used both for attenuation correction of the PET or SPECT images and for localization of the PET or SPECT image findings.
   (c) (a) and (b).

Answers

1. (c).

2. (c).

CHAPTER 11

Image Reconstruction, Processing, and Display

In the modern nuclear medicine clinic, computers are highly integrated into the clinical workflow. Software algorithms are responsible for the critical tasks of image reconstruction from projections, and the display of digital data on computer monitors. In addition, specialized software may be employed in the processing of data for such tasks as reformatting, filtering to enhance or de-emphasize certain features in the images, and rendering surfaces or calculating specialized projections.

Reconstruction

Reconstruction is the process of creating transaxial slices from projection views. There are two basic approaches to creating the transaxial slices: **filtered backprojection** and **iterative reconstruction**. Filtered backprojection, which in the past was the dominant method for nuclear medicine tomographic reconstruction and is still the mainstay of CT reconstruction, will be covered in depth in this chapter. Iterative reconstruction, now ubiquitous in SPECT and PET reconstruction algorithms and beginning to appear in the CT domain, is more computationally intensive. A brief introduction to iterative reconstruction will presented at the end of this section.

Filtered backprojection

The process of backprojection will be introduced here, followed by a discussion of filtering.

Backprojection

In backprojection, the data acquired by the camera are used to create multiple **transaxial slices**. Figure 11.1 is a representation of this process; the 10 projection views are cut into seven bands and shown pulled apart. The bands forming each view are then shown smeared along a radius, like the spokes of a wheel. It is this smearing back toward the center that gives us the term "backprojection." The smears of the middle bands (shown in dark gray) are seen in translucent gray.

A simplification of the processes of projection and backprojection is illustrated in Figures 11.2 and 11.3. Figure 11.2 is a representation of data obtained in the acquisition of projection views of a thin radioactive disk. In this figure, an imaginary grid is placed over the disk (Figure 11.2(a)), the disk is imaged (Figure 11.16(b)), and the counts for each pixel are recorded (Figure 11.2(c)). The counts in each of the cells of a column are summed and stored in an array (Figure 11.2(d)). In a similar manner, all of the rows are summed, and stored in an array of sums to the right of the matrix (Figure 11.2(e)).

During backprojection, the two arrays of projection data are used to recreate an image of the original disk. In the upper panel of Figure 11.3, the upper array is spread, or backprojected, across the columns of a blank matrix so that each of the values in any single column are identical. The array to the right of the matrix is backprojected across the rows, and these values are added cell by cell to

Essentials of Nuclear Medicine Physics and Instrumentation, Third Edition. Rachel A. Powsner, Matthew R. Palmer, and Edward R. Powsner.
© 2013 John Wiley & Sons, Ltd. Published 2013 by John Wiley & Sons, Ltd.

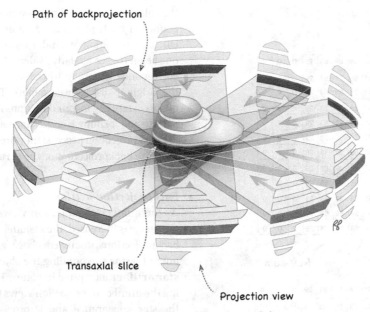

Figure 11.1 Projection views of a liver are backprojected to create transaxial slices.

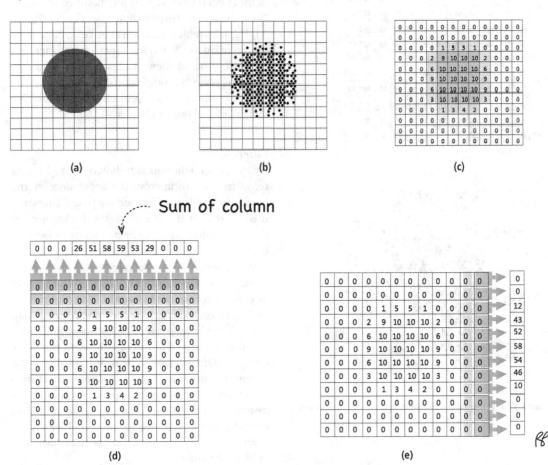

Figure 11.2 Acquisition of projection views (as numerical arrays) of a disk.

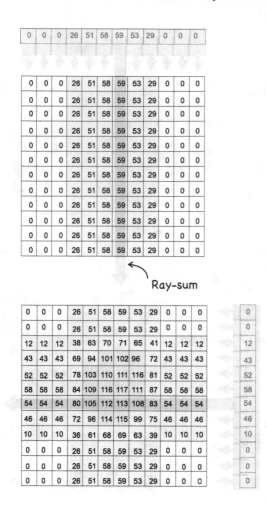

Ray-sum

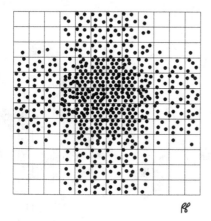

Figure 11.3 Projection views of a disk are backprojected.

the values of the preceding set (middle panel). If the counts in each pixel are represented by dots (for ease of illustration, each dot represents 5 counts), one begins to see a relatively dense central area that corresponds generally to the size and location of the original disk (lower panel). The wide bands of dots extending in four directions from this central density and forming a cross shape are an artifact of the backprojection process; they are residual counts from the backprojection of the arrays.

Backprojection artifact

As the number of projection views used to create the image is increased, the residual counts from the backprojections discussed above give the appearance of a star surrounding the object, the so-called **star artifact** illustrated in Figure 11.4(a). Increasing the number of projection views further removes the star appearance and improves the definition of the object (Figure 11.4(b), (c)); however, an overall "blur" remains surrounding the object (Figure 11.4(d)). This blur, which will be referred to from this point on as the **backprojection artifact**, is a demonstration of how backprojection does not really recreate the original object and is not the inverse of the process of projection (see Figure 7.4 and associated text in Chapter 7).

Filtering

Filtering is a mathematical technique applied during reconstruction to improve the appearance of the image. In particular, for our purposes, filters are used to reduce the effects of the backprojection ("blur") artifact and to remove image noise (see box).

When image data are represented in familiar terms, such as in counts per pixel, the data are said to exist in the **spatial domain**. Filtering can be performed on these data as they are. Alternatively, the data can be represented as a series of sine waves and the filtering performed on these. In the latter case, the data are said to be transformed into the **frequency domain**. Before we discuss this transformation of data from the spatial domain to the frequency domain, we shall apply some simple filters to data represented in the spatial domain in order to reduce the backprojection artifact and noise in the images.

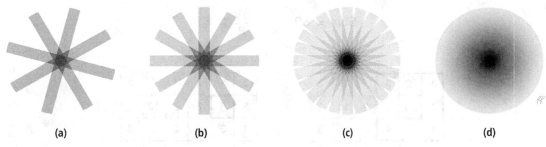

Figure 11.4 Star artifact and backprojection "blur" artifact.

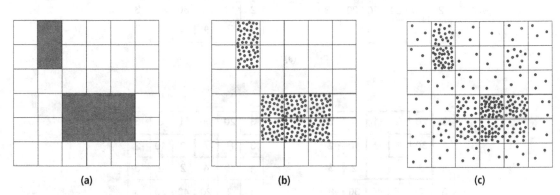

Figure 11.5 Statistical variation in counts.

Signal vs. Noise

The **signal** is that part of the information that produces the actual image; **noise** is extraneous data and may have no direct relation to the actual image. Noise reduces the quality of the image. Statistical variation in counts and random electronic fluctuations are among the sources of noise, which can be reduced by improved collimation, longer acquisition times, and better design of the circuitry.

Filtering in the spatial domain

Spatial Filtering to reduce noise: Nine-point smoothing: Figure 11.5 demonstrates the effects of noise on the images of two rectangles. In Figure 11.5(a), a grid is placed over the two rectangles being imaged. Figure 11.5(b) is a representation of an ideal image with uniformly distributed counts. Figure 11.5(c) is a more realistic representation of an acquired image of the rectangles. The counts are

greater over the rectangles than the background, but noise contributes to the inhomogeneity in the rectangles and the background.

Smoothing partially redistributes the counts from the pixels with the highest counts to their immediate neighbors; in this way, the more extreme irregularities in pixel counts are "blunted." The nine-point smoothing technique is demonstrated in Figure 11.6. The counts from the central pixel and eight immediately adjacent pixels are averaged (Figure 11.6(a)). The count in the central pixel is replaced by this average. This process is repeated pixel by pixel (Figure 11.6(b), (c)).

In one variation of this technique, the central pixel is given a different weight than its eight immediate neighbors. This smoothing filter is applied to pixel (2, 2) in Figure 11.7(a). The nine pixel elements centered on pixel (2, 2) are multiplied pixel by pixel by the corresponding elements in the so-called **filter kernel** (with a central weight of 10) as shown in Figure 11.7(b). The sum of all nine values in the resulting matrix (in this case 339) is divided by the sum of the nine elements of the filter kernel, 18. The resulting value, 19, is the filtered

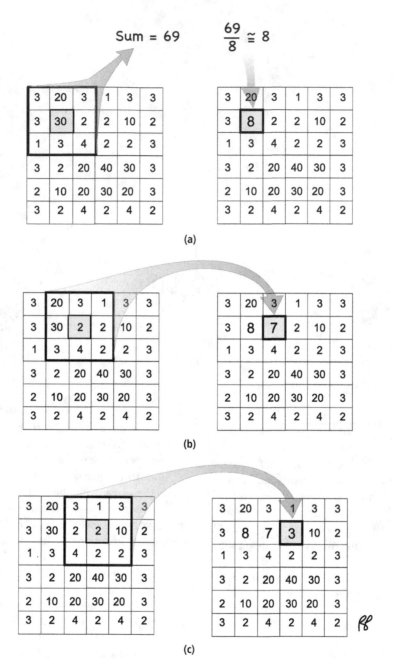

Figure 11.6 Nine-point smoothing.

value for pixel (2, 2) (Figure 11.7(c)). In this way, the original value of pixel (2, 2), 30, is modified by the influence of its nearest-neighbor pixels. This process is applied to each pixel of the matrix. The result of applying this process to each pixel in the matrix can be seen in Figure 11.8 (upper panel). If a kernel with a less heavily weighted central value of 2 is applied to the matrix, the final image is "more smoothed," that is, the edges of the rectangle are less distinct (lower panel).

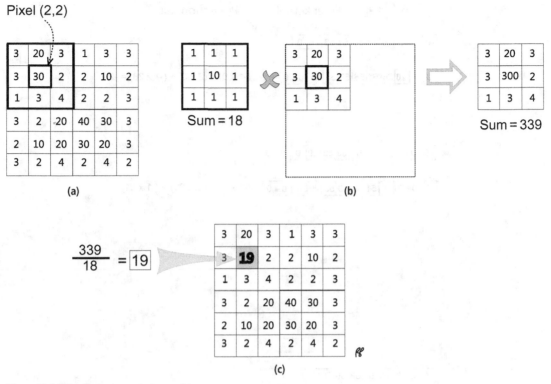

Figure 11.7 Weighted nine-point smoothing.

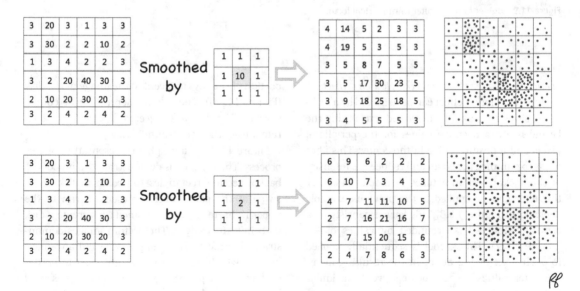

Figure 11.8 Nine-point smoothing using kernels with central weights of 10 and 2.

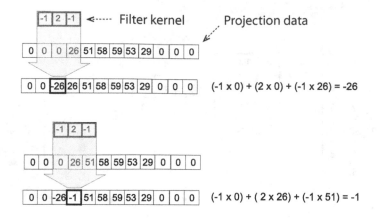

(-1 x 0) + (2 x 0) + (-1 x 26) = -26

(-1 x 0) + (2 x 26) + (-1 x 51) = -1

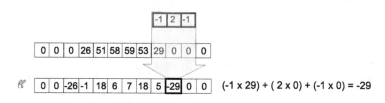

(-1 x 29) + (2 x 0) + (-1 x 0) = -29

Filtered data

Figure 11.9 Edge-enhancing filter in numerical form.

Spatial filtering to reduce the backprojection artifact: A somewhat different effect can be achieved by a technique similar to that just described, except that the kernel is given negative values for the peripheral pixels and a positive value in the center. This filter tends to enhance the edges and reduce the intensity of the backprojection artifact. A simple version of this filter can be applied to the previous example depicted in Figure 11.3. This kernel consists of a central value, +2, surrounded by values of −1 (Figure 11.9). This kernel is sequentially applied to each pixel of the array. In the resulting array, the outer values are zero or negative. In a similar fashion, the kernel is applied to the second array of the example in Figure 11.3. When these filtered arrays are backprojected, their peripheral negative values cancel counts in a manner that removes the

portion of the rays adjacent to the image of the disk (Figure 11.10). The relative depression of counts surrounding the backprojected disk helps to separate it from the background.

Figure 11.11 is a graphic representation of this process. The top panels demonstrate the process of backprojecting rectangles to create a disk. Each swipe of the paint roller represents a ray. In the upper right image, the combined rays create a disk with indistinct edges. The bottom images demonstrate the effects of a simple edge enhancement filter in which negative values are used to border each rectangle prior to backprojection (represented by the small white squares on either side of each rectangle). These negative values cancel contributions from adjacent ray-sums, and the circle's edge is seen more clearly (bottom right). The filter kernel

0	0	-26	-1	18	6	7	18	5	-29	0	0

0	0	-26	-1	18	6	7	18	5	-29	0	0		0
-12	-12	-38	-13	6	-6	-5	6	-7	-41	-12	2		-12
-19	-19	-45	-20	-1	-13	-12	-1	-14	-43	-19	-19		-19
12	24	-2	23	42	30	31	42	29	⁻5	12	12		24
3	3	-23	2	21	9	10	21	8	-26	3	3		3
10	10	-16	9	28	16	17	28	15	-19	10	10		10
4	4	-22	3	22	10	11	22	9	-25	4	5		4
28	28	2	27	46	34	35	46	33	-1	28	28		28
-26	-26	-48	-28	-8	-20	-19	8	-21	-55	-26	-26		-26
-10	-10	-36	-11	8	-4	-3	8	-5	-14	-10	-10		-10
0	0	-26	-1	18	6	7	18	5	-29	0	0		0
0	0	-26	-1	18	6	7	18	5	-29	0	0		0

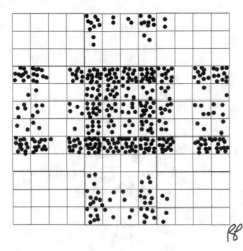

Figure 11.10 Backprojection following application of an edge-enhancing filter.

used here is similar to the kernel in the previous example.

Filtering in the frequency domain

Filtering in the spatial domain proves to be computationally burdensome. In general, it is easier to perform filtering in the frequency domain, once the data have been transformed. The following is meant to clarify this process.

Until this point, we have discussed data only in the most familiar terms, usually as counts per unit time or counts per pixel—in other words, in the **time domain** or in the **spatial domain**. We may

look at the data principally in terms of time, for example the 24 h uptake in the thyroid gland, or we may view an image of the spatial distribution of the activity in the thyroid. Although they serve different purposes, these two domains are not entirely independent. In fact, they only represent different views of the underlying data.

Now we propose to extend this concept of domains beyond the familiar ones of time and space to another—the **frequency domain**. In this rather unfamiliar domain, the distribution of counts across the image is expressed by a spectrum of spatial frequencies. The frequencies themselves are given in **cycles per centimeter** or **cycles per pixel**. This transformation of data facilitates the computations necessary for filtering.

The first step is the representation of an object as a sum of sinusoidal waves rather than as the arrangement of small dots that we usually refer to as an image in the spatial domain. Just as any sound pattern in air can be represented by a combination of sine and cosine waves given in cycles per second, any image pattern can be represented by a combination of sine and cosine waves in cycles per pixel. This use of sinusoidal waves to represent a simple object is illustrated in Figure 11.12. The original rectangles (seen in the top row of column (c)) can be plotted as a square wave (column (a)). A three-dimensional view of this square wave is drawn in column (b). Column (c) can be thought of as a bird's-eye view from the top of the three-dimensional square wave. The subsequent rows depict the process of the sequential addition of sine waves to approximate the square wave. The first sine wave (seen in column (a) in the second row) is a very rough approximation of the square wave, and when viewed from above poorly represents the original rectangles. A second sine wave (of higher frequency) is added to the first sine wave (shown in the third row). Each subsequent addition of a higher-frequency sine wave serves to sharpen the image of the rectangles in column (c).

In contrast to the original dot image, which can be described by the number of dots at each location, the amplitude of the wave at each frequency now describes the new image (Figure 11.13). This is the object (in our example, the two rectangles) described in the frequency domain, and a plot of amplitudes of the wave at each frequency is called its **frequency spectrum** (Figure 11.14). Amplitude, the height of

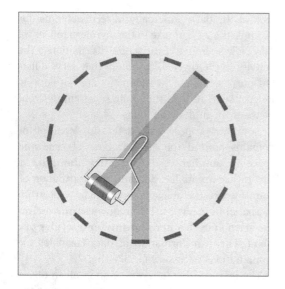
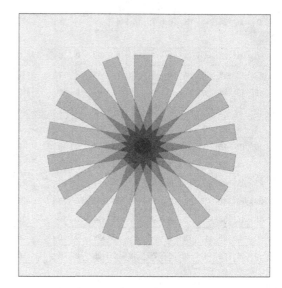
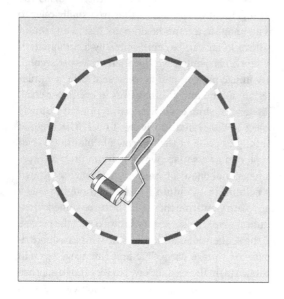
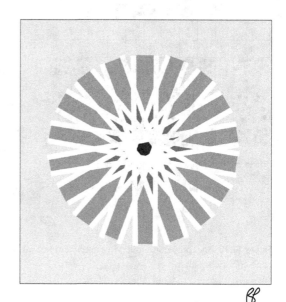

Figure 11.11 Graphic representation of an edge-enhancing filter.

the wave, is expressed in counts; frequency is measured in cycles per pixel.

The information obtained by the camera is not changed by this transformation of the collected data from the spatial to the frequency domain; all that is changed is the method of describing the data. More generally, we can say that data can be transformed from one domain into another with neither gain nor loss of the information contained.

Although we are interested here in mathematical methods of transforming data, it is worth mentioning that common physical devices, optical lenses for example, can also be used to transform data. The most pertinent data transformation from the spatial to the frequency domain is based on a method developed about 200 years ago by the French mathematician and physicist Joseph Fourier and is now referred to as the **Fourier transformation**. Its importance lies in the fact that very efficient algorithms are available for computing the Fourier transform, and so it saves time when filtering image data.

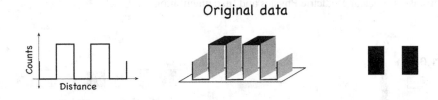

Original data

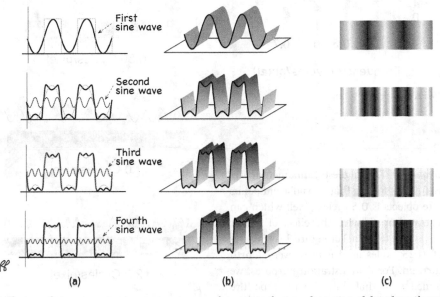

Sine wave approximation to original data

First sine wave

Second sine wave

Third sine wave

Fourth sine wave

(a)   (b)   (c)

Figure 11.12 The use of sine waves to represent an image: a key step in the transformation of data from the spatial to the frequency domain.

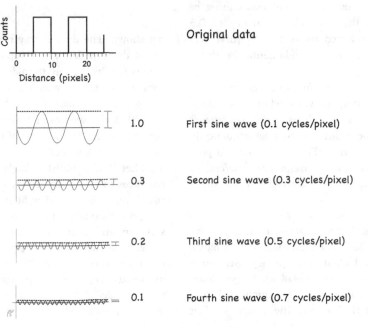

Original data

1.0   First sine wave (0.1 cycles/pixel)

0.3   Second sine wave (0.3 cycles/pixel)

0.2   Third sine wave (0.5 cycles/pixel)

0.1   Fourth sine wave (0.7 cycles/pixel)

Figure 11.13 Sine waves used to approximate the image of rectangles seen in Figure 11.12.

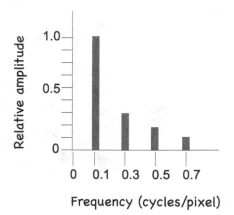

Figure 11.14 Frequency spectrum.

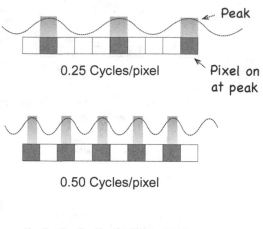

0.25 Cycles/pixel

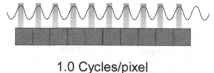

0.50 Cycles/pixel

1.0 Cycles/pixel

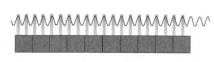

2.0 Cycles/pixel

Figure 11.15 The Nyquist frequency of 0.5 cycles/pixel is the smallest discernible frequency for a matrix.

Nyquist frequency: The highest fundamental frequency useful for showing that two adjacent points are separate objects is 0.5 cycles/pixel, which can be demonstrated by showing the effect of higher frequencies. In the top panel of Figure 11.15, a frequency of 0.25 cycles/pixel causes every fourth pixel to turn on. For demonstration purposes, we have assumed here that only the most positive portion of any sine wave can turn on a pixel. For a frequency of 0.5 cycles/pixel, every other pixel will be on. At still higher frequencies (1.0 cycles/pixel, 2.0 cycles/pixel, and so on), every pixel will be on; in this situation, one sine wave peak cannot be separated from the next. The frequency of 0.5 cycles/pixel is referred to as the **Nyquist frequency**; it is the highest fundamental frequency useful for imaging.

Although the Nyquist frequency is always 0.5 cycles/pixel, the numeric value when expressed in cycles/cm is a function of the pixel size. The smaller the pixel size, the greater the Nyquist frequency in cycles/cm. As shown in Figure 11.16, for a pixel size of 0.5 cm, 0.5 cycles/pixel is 1.0 cycle/cm; for a pixel size of 0.25 cm, it is 2 cycles/cm; and so on.

Signal, noise, and the backprojection artifact in the frequency domain: To understand the design of filters, it is necessary to look at the frequency distribution of the important components of an image. Figure 11.17(a) shows a distribution of frequencies derived from a hypothetical image; the image itself is

not shown. The darker gray bars derive from the signal data, which are composed principally of frequencies in the low to middle range; the white bars represent noise, which is nearly uniform across the spectrum. Following backprojection (Figure 11.17(b)), the spectra of both the signal and the noise are altered by the effect of the backprojection. In essence, backprojection acts as a kind of smoothing filter that diminishes higher frequencies and enhances the lower-frequency components of the signal and noise. An ideal filter would remove the backprojection artifact to restore the original signal spectrum and, at the same time, remove all of the noise. Unfortunately, the frequency ranges of the signal and noise overlap. The practical filters used in filtered backprojection operations are designed to make a trade-off between restoring the image detail and suppressing noise.

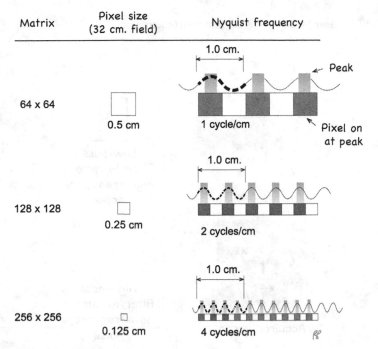

Matrix	Pixel size (32 cm. field)	Nyquist frequency

Figure 11.16 The Nyquist frequency expressed in cycles/cm.

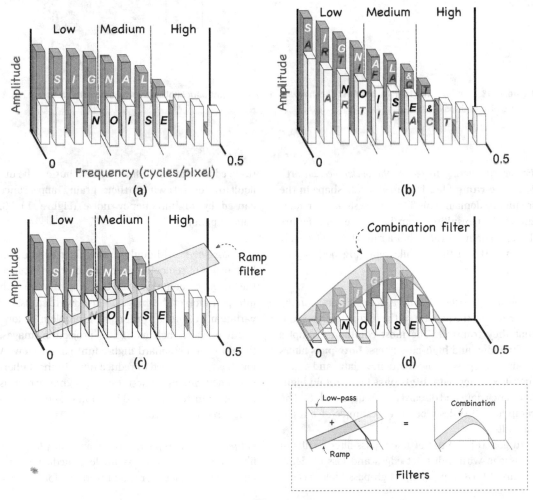

Figure 11.17 Effect of a ramp filter and a combination low-pass and ramp filter on signal data, statistical noise, and the backprojection artifact.

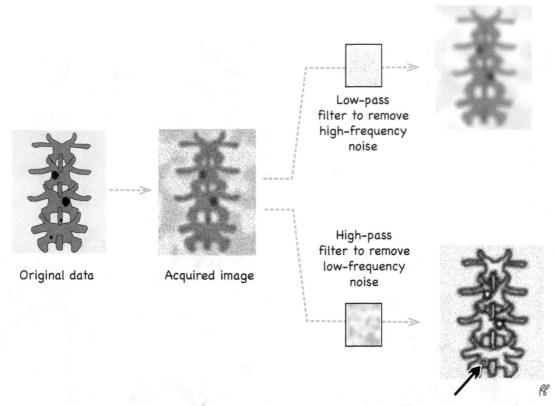

Figure 11.18 Low-pass and high-pass filters. The arrow in the lower right panel points to an image detail preserved by the use of a high-pass filter.

Frequency filtering to reduce the backprojection artifact: The **ramp** filter is named for its shape in the frequency domain. This filter was designed to reduce the artifact resulting from backprojection. Figure 11.17(c) demonstrates that a ramp filter effectively removes this artifact while retaining both signal and noise data.

Frequency filtering to reduce noise: Filters can be described by the portion of the frequency spectrum that they transmit. The most common examples are the low- and high-pass filters. **Low-pass** filters retain (or "pass") low-frequency data and reject high-frequency data; **high-pass** filters retain high-frequency data and discard low-frequency data. The ramp filter just described is an example of a high-pass filter.

In general, the use of a low-pass filter results in an image with indistinct edges and loss of detail (Figure 11.18, top panel). High-pass filters accen-

tuate edges and retain finer details, but can be difficult to interpret owing to their "grainy" appearance caused by high-frequency noise (Figure 11.18, bottom panel).

Low-pass filters: Although a ramp filter is an excellent means of removing the backprojection artifact, the image still contains noise that can interfere with interpretation of the images. Noise due to statistical variation in counts is more of a problem in low-count images, such as SPECT projection images, than it is in a standard high-count planar view. A low-pass filter is used to reduce noise in the higher-frequency ranges while retaining signal, which is predominantly composed of low- and middle-range-frequency data.

• *Types of low-pass filters:* There are many low-pass filters available to process nuclear medicine data, and all are named after their inventors, for example

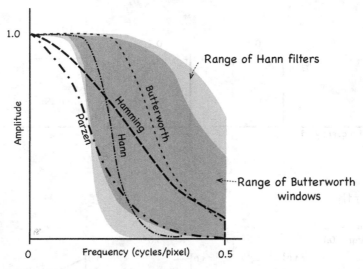

Figure 11.19 Characteristics of commonly used low-pass filters.

Hann (or von Hann), Hamming, Butterworth, Wiener, and Parzen. Each filter has a different shape (although some are quite similar), and when applied will modify the image differently.

Some typical low-pass filters used to reduce high-frequency noise are plotted in Figure 11.19. The Parzen filter is an example of a low-pass filter that greatly smooths data; generally it is not used for SPECT. The Hann and Hamming filters are low-pass filters with some smoothing but a relatively greater acceptance of mid- and high-frequency data than the Parzen filter. The commonly used Butterworth filter allows the user to adjust the relative degree of high-frequency wave acceptance (see below). The Butterworth and Hann filters are also "flexible" filters in that their shape can be altered by specifying certain parameters. The broad, light gray band in Figure 11.19 roughly delineates the possible range of shapes of the Hann filter; the darker gray band delineates the possible shapes of the Butterworth filter.

• *Cutoff Frequency and order:* The cutoff frequency, often referred to as the power of the filter, is the maximum frequency the filter will pass. If the cutoff frequency is greater than the Nyquist frequency, the filter is abruptly terminated at the Nyquist frequency of 0.5 cycles/pixel. A Hann filter with dif-

ferent cutoff frequencies is depicted in the upper panel of Figure 11.20. An additional parameter, the **order**, can be specified for Butterworth filters. The order controls the slope of the curve (lower panel of Figure 11.20).

Sequence for applying filters: Filters can be applied to the data prior to backprojection (**prefiltering**), during backprojection, or to the transaxial slices following backprojection. Often, the low-pass filters (Butterworth, Hann, Hamming, Parzen, and others) are applied as prefilters to remove high-frequency noise. A ramp filter is then applied during backprojection to remove the backprojection artifact. The prefilter and ramp filter can be applied in a single step (see Figure 11.17(d)). This **combination filter** is referred to either by the filter's name, for example "Parzen," or by a description such as "ramp–Parzen filter."

Filter selection: The selection of the optimal filter depends on both the characteristics of the data and the user's personal preference. In general, a high-pass filter is better suited for higher-count data, whereas a low-pass or smoothing filter is better for data containing a small number of counts. With respect to preference, some users like smoother, less detailed images; others are willing to tolerate the

Hann

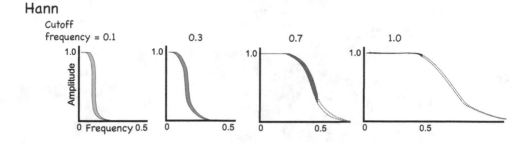

Butterworth

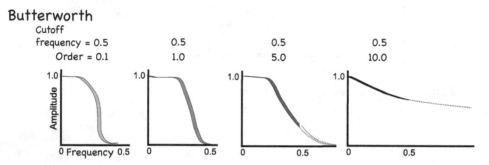

Figure 11.20 The Butterworth and Hann windows (or prefilters) can be modified to match the characteristics of the data set.

"grainy" appearance following the use of a high-pass filter in order to retain the finer details of the signal data.

Attenuation correction

Attenuation: Photons originating from inside the body are more likely to be absorbed or scattered by the surrounding tissue than photons originating near the surface. The attenuation coefficient for ^{99m}Tc in tissue (see Chapter 2) is 0.15/cm. This means that every centimeter of tissue between the source and camera will absorb or scatter approximately 15% of the photons entering. Attenuation of photons will reduce the counts from the middle of the body. In Figure 11.21, the photons from the deeper portions of the myocardium are less likely to exit the surface of the body than photons from the more superficial portions.

Attenuation correction: Attenuation correction was routinely performed in the past by calculation techniques that assumed a uniform tissue density across

the body and therefore uniform attenuation. Transmission imaging for measuring attenuation, which is rarely uniform across the body, has nearly completely replaced calculation techniques, especially for the chest, where densities corresponding to soft tissue, lung, and bone coexist in the same transaxial slices. However, calculated attenuation correction is still useful for brain imaging, where the consistency of the tissue is fairly uniform.

Calculated attenuation correction: Attenuation correction can be performed by applying a correction factor that takes into account the source depth and the tissue attenuation coefficient. The tissue attenuation coefficient is assumed to be a constant value throughout the cross section of the body.

There are several algorithms available for calculated attenuation correction. A simplified application of one such mathematical technique, the Chang algorithm, is the most commonly used method. Figure 11.22 highlights the major points of the method. An approximation to the outline of the head is drawn by computer or manually

(Figure 11.22(a)). Within the outline, a correction matrix is constructed; this is shown symbolically by shading (Figure 11.22(b)), in which the darker area indicates greater correction. As seen in Figure 11.22(c), the greater correction increases the number of counts in the deeper portions of the brain.

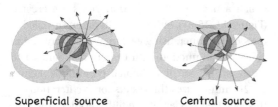

Superficial source   Central source

Figure 11.21 Attenuation of photons.

Transmission correction: In this technique, attenuation correction factors are obtained directly from **transmission** measurements. Transmission measurements are tomographic projections obtained from a radionuclide source positioned outside the patient on the side directly opposite the camera (Figure 11.23). The attenuation of photons through the body from this external source is dependent on the tissue thickness and the attenuation coefficient along the transmission rays. As the camera head and source are rotated around the patient, the attenuation of photons through the body between the source and the camera head varies. The transmission projections are used to correct emission projections prior to reconstruction. In hybrid imaging systems, such as PET-CT and SPECT-CT systems, the computed tomography (CT) data is used for attenuation correction and, as such, the rotating X-ray source can be thought of as a transmission

source. For these systems, a detector specifically designed for X-rays is a necessary addition. Attenuation correction using CT data is discussed in further detail in Chapter 8, and hybrid imaging systems are introduced in Chapter 10.

Iterative reconstruction
A relatively elegant technique called iterative reconstruction has steadily replaced filtered backprojection. Images reconstructed with this technique exhibit significantly less backprojection artifact (seen in Figure 11.4) than those created using filtered backprojection.

In iterative reconstruction, the computer starts with an initial "guess" estimate of the data to

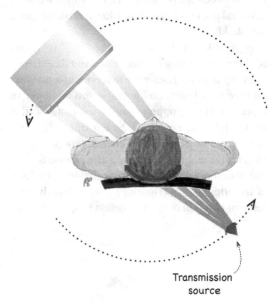

Transmission source

Figure 11.23 Transmission image.

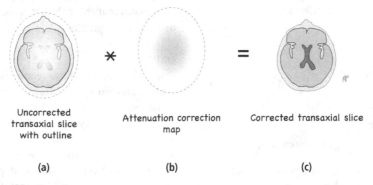

Uncorrected transaxial slice with outline

Attenuation correction map

Corrected transaxial slice

(a)   (b)   (c)

Figure 11.22 Attenuation correction.

produce a set of transaxial slices. These slices are then used to create a second set of projection views, which are compared with the original projection views as acquired from the patient. The transaxial slices from the computer's estimate are then modified using the difference between, or ratio of, the two sets of projection views. A new set of transaxial slices reconstructed from this modified, or second, estimate are then used to create a set of projection views, which are compared with the original projection views. Again these projection views are compared with the original projection views. If the process proceeds efficiently, each iteration generates a new set of projection views that more closely approximate the original projection views. The process is complete when the difference between the projection views of the estimated data and the original data is below a predetermined threshold.

Figures 11.24–11.26 are simplified illustrations of this process using a single transaxial slice shaped like a squared-off horseshoe to represent a transaxial slice of a heart, and a simple square object to represent the computer's initial estimate of this transaxial slice. Figure 11.24 illustrates the creation of the original and estimated data projection views. Figure 11.25 illustrates the comparison of the projection views for the first estimate with those of the original data (Figure 11.25(a)), and the subsequent creation of the correction projection views

from their ratio (Figure 11.25(b)). A transverse correction slice is then constructed by "backprojecting" these projection views (Figure 11.25(c)) (the correction slice and projection views are mathematical entities and, as such, are shaded in with an ambiguous pattern). The estimate of the first slice is then multiplied by this correction slice to create the second estimate slice (Figure 11.25(d)), from which a new set of projection views are created (Figure 11.25(e)). Subsequent iterations proceed in the same manner, using each new set of projection views in conjunction with the original data set to create a new set of estimated projections. Figure 11.26 summarizes the results for five iterations of this idealized model; at the fifth iteration, the estimated transaxial slice equals the original data and the process is complete.

In practice, most iterative reconstructions are terminated at a predetermined number of iterations, i.e., when the physician reading the studies is satisfied with the overall image quality, instead of allowing them to progress until the difference between the estimated and projection views reaches a set value. In general, the image resolution improves with increasing number of iterations, as demonstrated in Figure 11.27 using a single coronal slice of a lumbar spine from a SPECT bone scan. However, beyond a certain reasonable number of iterations, further improvements in resolution can only be accomplished at the cost of increased image noise.

Another advantage of iterative reconstruction compared with filtered backprojection is that corrections for attenuation, scatter, and even collimator and detector spatial resolution can be incorporated directly. The use of iterative reconstruction techniques was limited in the past because of lengthy computation times; faster computers and "shortcut" mathematical techniques such as OSEM have mitigated this problem.

OSEM

One widely used iterative reconstruction technique is the **maximum likelihood expectation maximization** (MLEM) algorithm. The computation time is very lengthy when all of the projection views are used in each iteration to create the correction slices. To shorten the processing time, a smaller group, or **subset**, of matched projection views from the estimated and original datasets are used

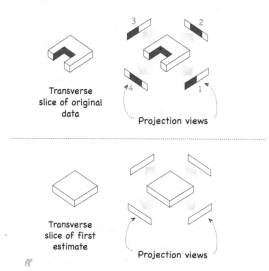

Figure 11.24 Simplified "projection" views of original and computer-estimated transaxial slices.

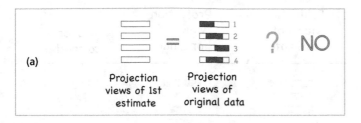

(a)

Projection views of 1st estimate   Projection views of original data

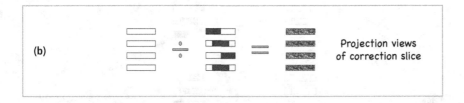

(b)

Projection views of correction slice

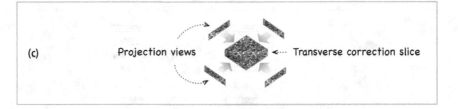

(c)   Projection views   Transverse correction slice

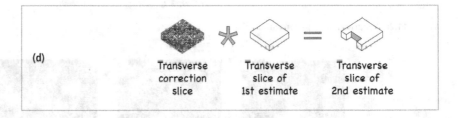

(d)

Transverse correction slice   Transverse slice of 1st estimate   Transverse slice of 2nd estimate

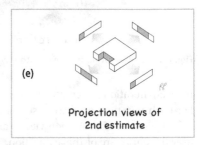

(e)

Projection views of 2nd estimate

Figure 11.25 (a) Projection views from the first estimate are compared with the projection views from the original data. Note that the projection views are oriented as seen by an outside observer looking toward the transaxial slice of the original data shown in Figure 11.24. (b) Correction projection views. (c) Transverse correction slice. (d) Second-estimate transverse slice. (e) Second-estimate projection views.

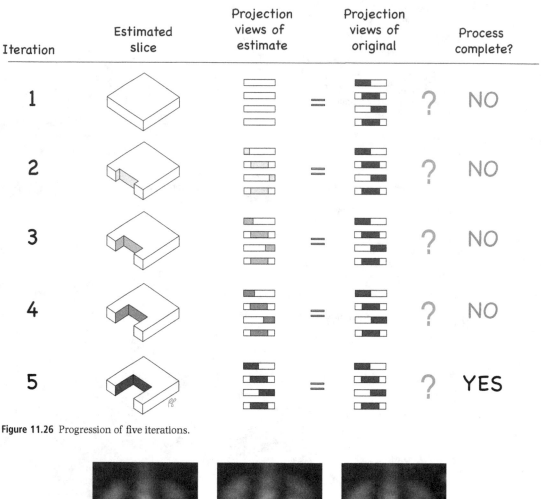

Figure 11.26 Progression of five iterations.

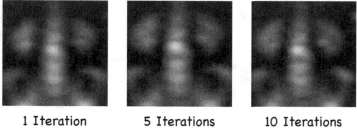

1 Iteration   5 Iterations   10 Iterations

Figure 11.27 Resolution improves with increasing number of iterations.

in each iteration to create the correction slices. For each iteration, a different subset is used. Each subset consists of projection views sampled evenly over the entire arc of the acquisition, 180 or 360°. For example, the first subset might contain every 12th projection view, beginning with the first projection view. The second subset might contain every 12th projection view, beginning with the sixth projection view, and so on. The process of using subsets for expectation maximization is called **ordered subsets expectation maximization (OSEM).**

Postreconstruction image processing

Multiplanar reformatting

Stacks of transverse images can be resliced or resampled in a process called multiplanar reformatting. From these reconstructed transverse images, **sagittal, coronal,** and oblique views can be generated. By convention, transaxial slices are oriented perpendicular to the long axis of the body. Sagittal and coronal slices are oriented parallel to the long axis of the body and at right angles to each other (Figure

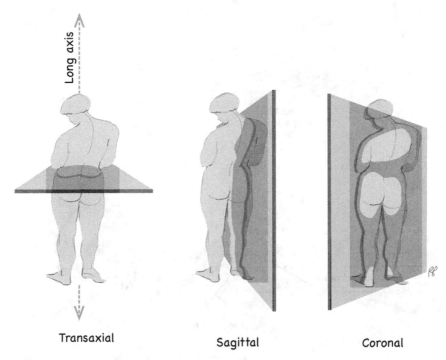

Long axis

Transaxial   Sagittal   Coronal

Figure 11.28 Transaxial, sagittal, and coronal images.

11.28). In a similar way, the axes of the heart are defined relative to the heart's long axis, understood to be the line running from base to apex. The **horizontal long axis view** and **vertical long axis view** are oriented parallel to the long axis of the heart. The **short axis view** is oriented perpendicular to the long axis of the heart (Figure 11.29). Multiplanar reformatted sliced images can be computed and saved in the computer or can be produced live, at the time of display.

Why reformatting works

Cross-sectional nuclear medicine image data acquired with SPECT or PET scanners typically have what are referred to as cubic or near-cubic **voxels** (voxels are the three-dimensional equivalent of two-dimensional pixels). A cubic voxel means that each side of the voxel is identical in length. As a result, the spatial resolution in all three planes (axial, sagittal, and coronal) is identical. Therefore the stored image data can be sliced in any of the planes and retain consistent distances between points.

Advanced display techniques

Contrast enhancement

X-ray CT and some nuclear medicine images possess information over such a range of intensities that they cannot be displayed so that a human observer can see the intensity variations in the brightest and darkest portions of the image. This property of the image is referred to as **dynamic range**—formally defined as the ratio between the largest and smallest possible intensity changes. Display monitors are usually set up to display 256 intensities (gray levels), and the mathematical operation of mapping the image values (perhaps thousands of intensities) onto the 256-level scale is known as contrast manipulation or **contrast enhancement** (not to be confused with the other common use of this phrase in reference to the use of injected or ingested contrast materials for enhancing characteristics of anatomy during CT imaging). Contrast enhancement schemes can be quite sophisticated, such as a mapping that exaggerates the differences between the darkest objects in an image and diminishes the differences between the brightest objects in the image. Another approach to contrast enhancement

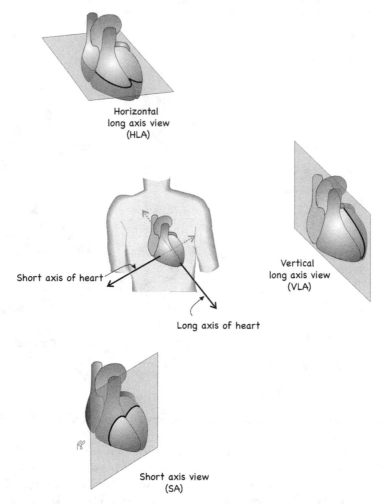

Horizontal
long axis view
(HLA)

Vertical
long axis view
(VLA)

Short axis of heart

Long axis of heart

Short axis view
(SA)

Figure 11.29 Oblique views of the heart.

involves compressing the broad range of intensities in the entire image to fit into 256 levels. One can also expand the scale to cut off low and high intensities, such that anything below a certain value appears black and anything above another value appears white. This latter scheme is referred to in radiology as **windowing** (not to be confused with windowing in the filtering sense), where the mapping of contrast is defined by a window level—the data intensity value that will be assigned to 128 (half-intensity)—and the window width—the range of data intensities that fill the displayed brightness scale.

As discussed in Chapter 9, each pixel of a CT image can be assigned a value in Hounsfield units, which ranges from −1000 HU (air) to greater than 1000 (dense cortical bone). Portions of the dynamic range from −1000 to 1000 are mapped onto the 0

to 256 range of the display monitor. This greatly improves the image contrast for the type of tissue of interest. For example, selecting "lung windows" on the workstation might set the window level to −500 and the width to 1500, and "bone windows" might set the level to 500 and the width to 2000. These selections center the displayed intensity in the mid-range for the expected or typical CT number in that anatomical feature, i.e., −500 for lung features and 500 for bone features, and then set a window width that preserves a broad range of intensities. Alternatively, the interpreter might select "liver windows," with a level of 95 and a width of only 100, thereby amplifying small intensity changes above and below the expected intensity in the liver. The three most commonly used windows, for soft tissue, lung, and bone, are depicted in Figure 11.30.

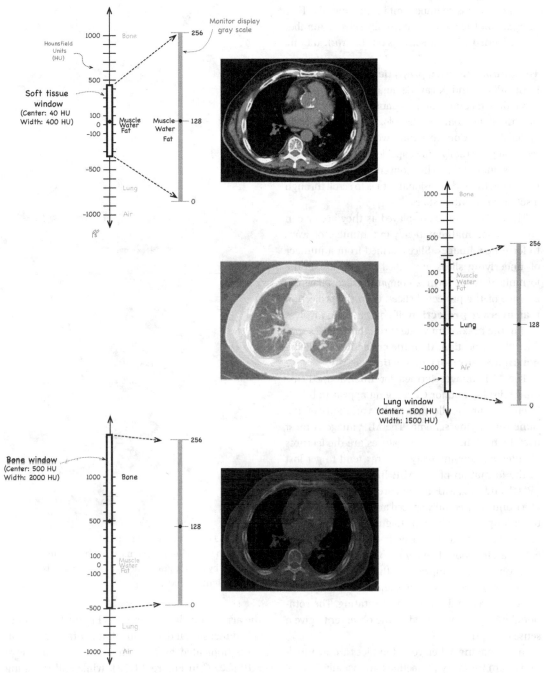

Figure 11.30 CT image contrast enhancement using variable windowing based on Hounsfield unit values. A standard range of Hounsfield unit values used to display soft tissue with a sample transaxial slice is shown at the top; ranges and images for lung and bone are shown in the middle and bottom, respectively.

Windowing is so important in the analysis of CT images that the viewer can usually select a number of predefined window settings on the workstation.

Maximum intensity projections

Both SPECT and X-ray CT image data are called three-dimensional data because they represent underlying anatomy or physiology over three spatial dimensions. Conventional workstation display technology is really only capable of displaying two-dimensional data. The conventional method of rendering three-dimensional data is to scroll through a set of consecutive slices.

These slices can be displayed as they are or can be combined mathematically in a number of ways to form new images. Slices formed from a number of underlying slices are called projections. If the formula used to form a computed slice takes the average of the projected slices, then the projection is an **average projection**. If computation involves taking the maximum value through the slices that form the projection, then the projection is called a **maximum intensity projection**, or MIP.

The MIP images formed for nuclear medicine image display and for CT imaging appear to be different but are really just slight variations of the same underlying scheme. The MIP image is most useful when the brightest features are the features of interest. Low-intensity features tend to get lost in the formation of the MIP. In nuclear medicine SPECT and PET, MIP images are usually computed at a number of equally spaced angles perpendicular to the long axis of the body (Figure 11.31) and then played back as a movie or a dynamic sequence called a cine-loop. In playing back the views, the observer has the impression that anatomical features are suspended in a somewhat transparent three-dimensional space that is rotating. The rotational motion is processed by the observer to give a sense of depth.

In CT imaging, when very thin slices are acquired, maximum intensity projections are usually formed by processing groups of consecutive slices. Again, this is most useful in applications where the most intense features in images are of most interest, for example when intravenous contrast is used for imaging, or in cases where small details seen in only one slice would be lost by averaging information over several slices. The MIP collapses the most intense features of individual slices (indicated by

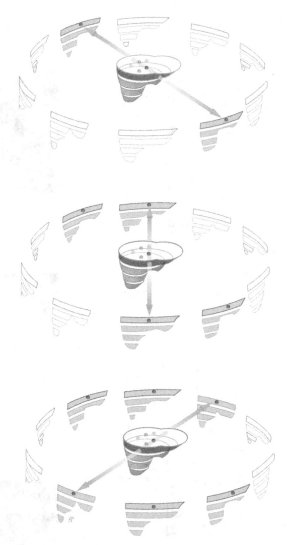

Figure 11.31 Nuclear medicine maximum intensity projection (MIP) image. The most intense feature (depicted by a dark gray sphere) along any ray is projected onto the MIP image.

the arrows on slices A and B in Figure 11.32) onto two-dimensional depictions that contain these features (indicated by the arrows on the transverse MIP slice C in Figure 11.32), while still retaining some anatomical detail. Figure 11.33 demonstrates how a small pulmonary nodule is accentuated in a CT MIP image compared with an average intensity projection image.

Surface and volume rendering

Other types of three-dimensional displays of SPECT or CT data can be used to enhance presentation and

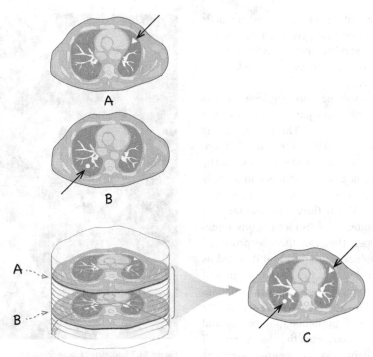

Figure 11.32 The MIP CT image collapses the most intense features from several sequential slices into a single image.

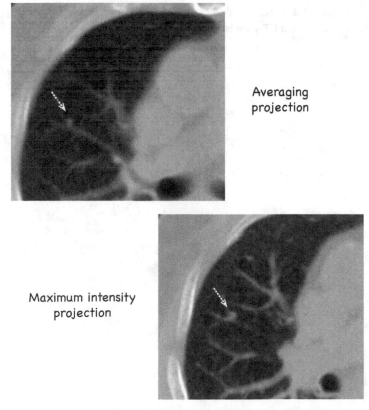

Averaging
projection

Maximum intensity
projection

Figure 11.33 The MIP image for a lung CT image accentuates image detail.

can aid in interpretation. Two standard methods of display, surface rendering (visualization of the surface of the data) and volume rendering (a more transparent view of the data set), are available on many workstations.

Both surface and volume rendering depend on, as the first step, the ability to segment the image data into multiple separate regions. This process is performed automatically and works best when image features are easily classified by intensity. Such is the case, for example, for bony structures and airways in CT and for specific lesions or tracer-avid anatomy in SPECT images. When three-dimensional data have been segregated into distinct regions representing tissue types, they can then be processed by computer graphics algorithms and depicted as virtual scenes. In this step, the tissues are treated as though they have real-world optical qualities such as color and texture. The graphics rendering assumes a position of an illumination source and computationally recreates what the observer would see, by tracing light rays transmitted from the source and reflected off a surface model or transmitted through and attenuated by portions of a volume model. An example of a surface rendering of a portion of the skeleton from a CT scan is seen in Figure 11.34.

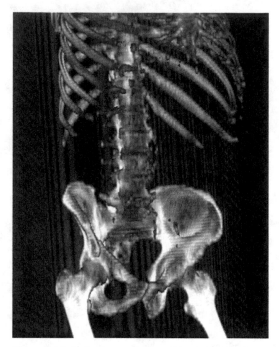

Figure 11.34 Skeletal tissue from a CT scan displayed using surface rendering.

Questions

1. Which of the following statements about the filtering used in reconstruction is correct?
   (a) Filtering is used to reduce noise and preserve signal data in the image.
   (b) Filtering cannot be applied to the data prior to backprojection.
   (c) Filtering is used to reduce artifacts created during backprojection.

2. True or false: The frequency domain represents an image as a sum of sine waves.

3. Match the following statements with either "low-pass filter" or "high-pass filter":
   (a) Used to remove high-frequency noise such as noise from statistical variation in counts.
   (b) Used to remove the "blur" from the backprojection artifact.
   (c) Can create "grainy" images, but preserves detail.
   (d) Creates "smoother" images, but image detail may be lost.

4. Which of the following statements about filters is correct?
   (a) The Nyquist frequency is 5.0 cycles/pixel.
   (b) The cutoff frequency of a filter is the minimum frequency the filter will pass.
   (c) Nyquist filters have an additional parameter called the order of the filter, which controls the slope of the curve.
   (d) All of the above.
   (e) None of the above.

5. Which of the following statements are true about iterative reconstruction?
   (a) Images reconstructed with iterative reconstruction have less backprojection artifact than those reconstructed with filtered backprojection.
   (b) Attenuation correction can be applied during iterative reconstruction.

   (c) Owing to long computational times, "shortcut" techniques such as ordered subsets expectation maximization are often used in iterative reconstruction.
   (d) Successive iterations are performed until the projection views of the estimate closely approximate the original data or until a predefined number of iterations have been completed.
   (e) All of the above.
   (f) None of the above.

6. To correct for attenuation effects in SPECT imaging with ^{99m}Tc, the correction matrix might be based upon:
   (a) The attenuation coefficient for 140 keV photons in Pb (lead).
   (b) The transmission from a single-photon-emission radionuclide source.
   (c) The known attenuation coefficient for 140 keV photons in tissue.
   (d) Transmission from a PET transmission source.
   (e) Transmission from an X-ray beam.

7. True or false: Measured tissue attenuation using transmission sources is generally more accurate than calculation techniques for attenuation correction for the thorax.

8. True or false: MIP (maximum intensity projection) images for SPECT and PET are used to accentuate the brightest details in a study.

9. Windowing is important in CT imaging because:
   (a) The range of pixel values in a CT image is much greater than the 256-level gray scale range available on a computer monitor.
   (b) The range of X-ray energies used to create the images must be reduced in order to see detail.
   (c) Only a small section of a CT image can be viewed at one time.

Answers

1. (a) and (c). Filtering can be applied before, during, and after backprojection, so (b) is incorrect.
2. True.
3. (a) Low-pass filter. (b) High-pass filter. (c) High-pass filter. (d) Low-pass filter.
4. (e). The Nyquist frequency is 0.5 cycles/pixel, the cutoff frequency refers to the maximum fre-quency the filter will pass, and the Butterworth filters have an additional parameter called the order of the filter.
5. (e).
6. (b), (c), (e).
7. True.
8. True.
9. (a).

CHAPTER 12

Information Technology

Just as we encounter, every day in our world, resources that are increasingly interconnected by an electronic infrastructure, so has the radiology and nuclear medicine environment evolved. Imaging devices are no longer stand-alone pieces of equipment but now operate as intelligent nodes in a networked environment. A sample networked radiology environment is shown in Figure 12.1.

Network

Imaging devices, workstations, and computers are connected within a hospital or department over a **local area network** (LAN) using a set of standards built upon Ethernet communications. The basis of Ethernet communications is that communicating devices share a common medium for communication and that data is broken up into packets that are sent out over the network and then reassembled at the destination. When a device wishes to send an information packet to another device, it essentially attaches an address to the data and sends it out on the network. The network takes care of routing it to the destination, whether it is across the room or across the world.

For a number of reasons to do with security and efficiency, rather than the entire world (or **wide-area network**, WAN) communicating on the same medium, the Ethernet is organized as a set of interconnected local area networks (LANs). Data flows unimpeded between nodes of the same LAN but must go through a gateway when it needs to be delivered to another LAN or to the WAN. In addition, the gateway might perform some security

operations, for example to make certain destinations inaccessible or to block certain types of communications from entering the LAN. This is particularly important in a hospital environment, where images and patient-related data must be protected from being accessible to people beyond those directly involved in patient care. In fact, when information flows on the WAN, there is no way to control what other machines do with it. Therefore, if images or data were to be sent out over the network, even if the destination was a trusted computer, for example in a referring doctor's office, there would be no way to ensure that a copy had not been made by one of the machines that was involved in routing the packets.

As the utility of a broadly connected network architecture has grown over the years, the issues associated with security and protecting data have become more pressing. It is not uncommon in hospital environments to need to connect imaging equipment at a remote location into the clinic's LAN structure. One example of this situation might be when a SPECT camera is located at a remote clinic. Another example might involve the diagnostic workstations used during holidays and off-hours for performing emergency image interpretation. In both situations, you have two LANs that must be connected over the public WAN while maintaining a secure environment. The technology for this structure is referred to as a **virtual private network** (VPN). Software operating on both LANs intercepts all the traffic and encrypts it for communication before it is released onto the public Internet. This way, even if an unauthorized computer

Essentials of Nuclear Medicine Physics and Instrumentation, Third Edition. Rachel A. Powsner, Matthew R. Palmer, and Edward R. Powsner.
© 2013 John Wiley & Sons, Ltd. Published 2013 by John Wiley & Sons, Ltd.

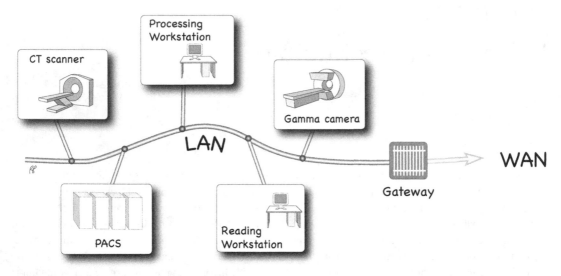

Figure 12.1 Simplified network diagram for a radiology department.

were to make a copy of the data during transit, the data would be nonsensical without access to the encryption details.

DICOM

Most modern diagnostic imaging devices are now built to communicate using a standard referred to as DICOM (Digital Imaging and Communications in Medicine). The DICOM standard is a set of rules that establishes the manner in which image data is transmitted from one machine to another, and also imposes a structure on the radiological data. A **DICOM information object** consists of image data and associated information such as, for example, patient name, date of birth, and time of acquisition. The nonimage portion of the DICOM data is often referred to as the "header," the pieces of information are "fields," and these fields have names that are referred to as "tags." The tag names are generally descriptive. For example, the patient's date of birth is stored as an eight-character sequence representing year, month, and day in a DICOM field with the tag name "PatientBirthDate." A diagram representing a DICOM information object is shown in Figure 12.2.

The DICOM image and header data are packaged for communication or storage in a manner such that they cannot be easily separated. A single

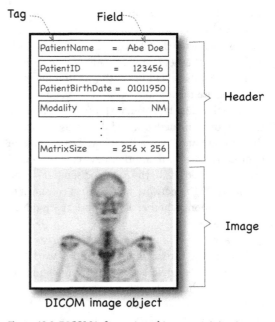

Figure 12.2 DICOM information object, containing image and header.

DICOM object contains a large and variable number of header tags but only one image—say, one radiographic view or one slice from a multislice CT scan, although this image can have multiple frames. In nuclear medicine studies packaged as DICOM objects, it is common to use a multiframe format to encode a sequence of projections from a SPECT study or a sequence of frames recorded in a dynamic study.

Many of the DICOM header tags are common to all examination types. Some examples of such fields are the patient name (PatientName), date of birth (PatientBirthDate), and the name of the institution where the examination was performed (InstitutionName). Other tags are modality-specific, such as the kVp (KVP) and mA (XrayTubeCurrent) of a CT scan. The modality itself is coded as a two-letter sequence in the Modality tag. The modality codes for CT, PET, and nuclear medicine are CT, PT, and NM, respectively. DICOM-compliant devices can generally understand the structure of and store or send DICOM information objects regardless of modality, but do not need to be capable of interpreting each object. For example, a particular display workstation might be able to receive and display planar X-rays and slices from a CT examination and receive PET images, but might not be able to display PET images correctly.

DICOM is, strictly speaking, a communications protocol that has evolved to also function as a universal storage format. Its adoption by all the major vendors of medical imaging devices has helped to impose a uniform structure on how a radiological examination is structured. In DICOM terminology, medical images are grouped into one or more **series**, which are then grouped together as a **study**. Studies and series have unique identifiers (UIDs), which consist of a long sequence of numerals. Study, series, and image UIDs are generated by the scanner at the time of creation in such a way as to be globally unique. They are never reused and they can never be duplicated by any other scanner in the world. Studies and series usually have names (StudyDescription, SeriesDescription), which are either chosen at the discretion of the technologist or selected from a standard set used in an institution. An example of this type of hierarchical organization is shown in Figure 12.3. In this examination, the study is a SPECT-CT parathyroid scan that consists of four series with the series descriptions "Ant Pinhole," "Transverse NM," "Transaxial CT," and "Fused Transverse." Each series contains one or more DICOM image objects. By convention, as discussed above, the transverse slices from the SPECT scan are stored as a single multiframe DICOM image object, whereas each transaxial CT slice and each

transverse fused slice are stored as individual DICOM image objects.

PACS

At the heart of the modern electronic radiology or nuclear medicine clinic is a **picture archiving and communications system** (PACS). The PACS in a large radiology department can consist of a large number of computers with various specialized roles, or it could be just a single computer attached to the network that communicates information between a few imaging devices and workstations. One of the central roles of the PACS is the storage of image data, and in this respect it is the functional equivalent of what used to be the film archive. Image information is stored in the PACS archive, usually on hard disk drives but also on various types of media such as DVDs.

In general, the DICOM format is used for PACS storage and communication. This enhances the compatibility of the various systems, since modality computers, workstations, and various other imaging components generally have DICOM capabilities. This may not be the case throughout the system, however, as vendor-specific formats and protocols might be used to gain a speed advantage or to compress data for storage.

The set of networked computers and associated software that comprises the PACS might also have various other capabilities. It is common in modern hospital environments for the PACS to be capable of transferring image data to CDs or DVDs that can then be sent to referring doctors or given to patients. In addition, there is sometimes a need to print hard copy (paper, photographic paper, or maybe film) of images that reside in the PACS archive. The computers used by radiologists for diagnostic readout and by technologists for management and quality control purposes are also often considered to be part of the PACS infrastructure. And, finally, many PACS networks have the ability to modify their images in such a way that they can be viewed with a standard Web browser or with a simple piece of software referred to as a thin client.

Information systems

The modern electronic clinic needs to communicate not just image information but also information to

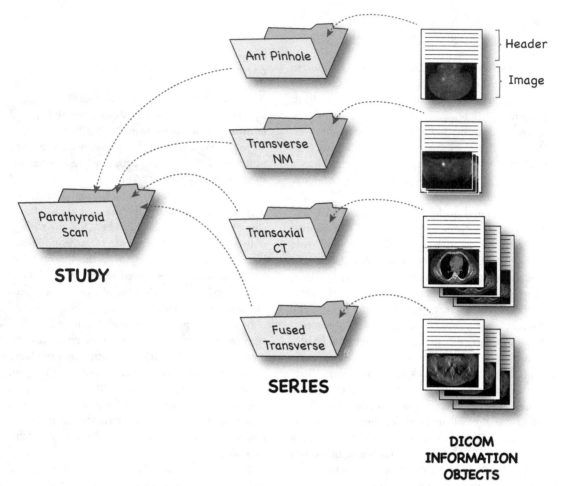

Figure 12.3 DICOM objects are grouped in series, which are then grouped together into studies.

assist the clinical workflow. Radiology reports and scheduling and billing procedures are examples of electronic information that is not part of the image object and for which there are no DICOM capabilities. The management and communication of this type of information is the job of the **radiology information system** (RIS). The RIS computers are also connected via the network and use a language called HL7 to code the information.

Other departments in the hospital, such as pathology departments and various clinics, are also typically highly integrated and dependent on digital information and computer communication. The collection of computers that manage information at the hospital level and communicate with the RIS and department-level information systems are

referred to as the **hospital information system** (HIS).

Information systems for hospital environments are developed in a highly dynamic milieu. The exact information responsibilities of the HIS, RIS, and PACS are not well defined or "nailed down" by standards and so they vary by vendor and product. An international collaboration known as **Integrating the Healthcare Environment** (IHE) is an effort to promote standardization for information sharing within the hospital environment. IHE has representation from governments, industry, and professional organizations and, in particular, from the radiology and nuclear medicine community. Standardization of information sharing will facilitate communication between components of

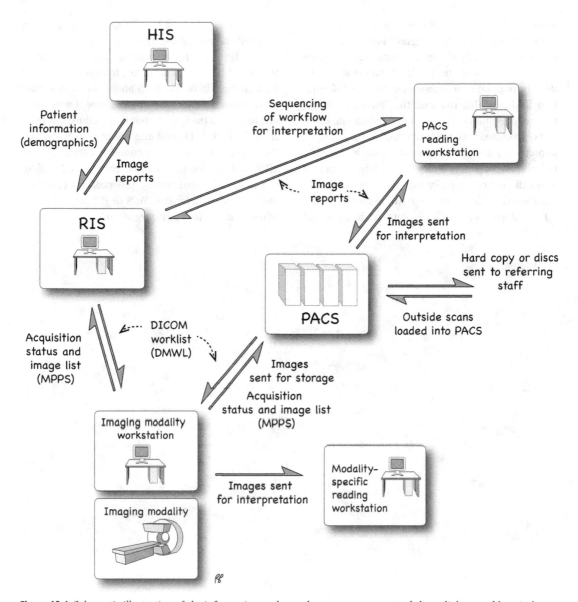

Figure 12.4 Schematic illustration of the information exchange between components of the radiology and hospital computer systems.

the information systems within hospitals while reducing the need for extensive local customization.

Figure 12.4 shows a sample topology for a radiology department working within an HIS/RIS environment.

Additional DICOM capabilities

There are two DICOM functions that are not really integral to the coding and communication of image

data but are important for facilitating the flow of information between modalities, the PACS, and the HIS/RIS. These are the **DICOM modality worklist** (DMWL) and the **modality performed procedure step** (MPPS). The associated structure and protocols are defined as part of the DICOM standard.

A **worklist server** is a computer on the network that obtains scheduling and demographic information from RIS and sends this information out in the form of DMWL messages to modality workstations in response to "worklist queries." From these messages, the modality computer obtains an accurate set of patient- and study-related data that can be used to populate the subsequent DICOM information fields. In this manner, the DMWL messages ensure information precision and reduce the problems associated with mistaken entries. For example, in preparing a scanner for a patient study, the technologist might simply query the worklist server and select the next patient by name or medical record number. The DMWL message would then transmit other information such as date of birth, exact patient name, various control numbers, the exact name of the procedure, and so on.

The MPPS, on the other hand, provides a way for the modality-related computers to pass information back to the RIS or the PACS about progress within a study. Essentially, there are two types of messages, one to inform the system that a procedure has been started (N-CREATE) and another to convey the fact that a procedure has been completed (N-SET). The MPPS completion message also contains a list of all the images created during the procedure, which makes it possible for the PACS or RIS to determine whether it received a complete study.

Questions

1. A physician in California wants to send SPECT images across the country to her colleague in Massachusetts for a second opinion on a case. To ensure privacy, she could do which of the following?

   (a) Send a CD containing the images using a trusted courier service.

   (b) Attach snapshots of the images to an e-mail.

   (c) Upload snapshots of the images to a Web-based picture-sharing service and simply not tell anyone else except the physician colleague how to access the images.

   (d) Send DICOM images using a VPN that was set up by IT departments in the two institutions.

2. If a DICOM worklist server computer is temporarily not functioning correctly, which of the following scenarios might ensue and have an impact on the clinic?

   (a) Packets get lost or routed incorrectly, and drop-out artifacts may appear in the images.

   (b) Patient scheduling information will not be available, and so the front-office staff cannot book future appointments.

   (c) Technologists will have to enter patient information manually in the modality work-station computers and may make typographical errors that will need to be fixed at a later time.

   (d) The record of which studies were performed will be lost, and so billing information will have to be entered manually.

3. When a physician is accessing a SPECT-CT study on the PACS system, he encounters some missing CT slices. Which of the following is the likely cause and potential solution?

   (a) The CT scanner likely stopped collecting data for a brief period during the study. Put the patient back into the scanner and reacquire the study.

   (b) The PACS workstation that the physician is using is probably faulty. The physician should log in to another workstation and re-access the study.

   (c) Owing to a network error, some CT slices were lost when the study was transmitted from the modality workstation to the PACS system. Retransmit the study.

   (d) There may be simply a delay somewhere in the system. Wait for five minutes and then try to access the study again on the PACS.

Answers

1. (a) and (d). E-mail is not generally secure and could be intercepted by a third party. Web-based photo- or picture-sharing sites are not generally secure, even if it seems unlikely that a third party would view the images.

2. (c). The worklist server communicates patient demographics from the RIS or HIS and avoids errors associated with manual entry.

3. (c) is the most likely. (d) is possible—in a congested network environment and with complicated transfers of large amounts of data between multiple computers, it is possible to accumulate significant delays.

CHAPTER 13

Quality Control

To ensure dependable performance of equipment, every nuclear medicine department is required to perform a routine series of tests on each device. These tests comprise the quality control program for the department.

Nonimaging devices

Dose calibrator

The testing performed on dose calibrators is quite rigorous, to ensure that correct radiopharmaceutical doses are administered to patients. Dose calibrators are checked for accuracy, constancy, linearity, and geometry.

Accuracy

Accuracy is a measure of the readings of the dose calibrator in comparison with well-accepted standards. Two long-lived nuclide sources, such as ^{137}Cs (half-life = 30 years) and ^{57}Co (half-life = 270 days), are measured repeatedly in the calibrator and the average readings are compared with values issued by the National Institute of Standards and Technology (NIST) for that particular source. If the readings differ from the standards by more than 10%, the dose calibrator should not be used. Accuracy should be checked at *installation*, *annually*, and *after repairs* or *when the instrument is moved* to a new location within the clinic.

Constancy

To ensure that the calibrator readings are constant from day to day, a long-lived nuclide such as ^{137}Cs is measured in the dose calibrator. The reading should not vary by more than 10% from the value

recorded in the initial accuracy test, corrected for the decay of the ^{137}Cs standard. The readings at each predefined setting (or "channel")—^{99m}Tc, ^{131}I, ^{67}Ga, etc.—are recorded and compared with previous readings. **Constancy** testing (including the channel checks) is performed *daily*.

Linearity

Linearity tests the calibrator over the range of doses used, from the highest dose administered to a patient down to approximately 5 µCi. One method of checking linearity is to measure a sample with the maximum activity that a department will use, such as 7.4 GBq (200 mCi) of ^{99m}Tc, and to repeat the measurement at regular intervals such as 6, 24, 30, and 48, and 96 h. A more rapid technique is to measure the dose unshielded, and then repeat the measurement of the same dose shielded within **lead sleeves** of varying thickness. The thicknesses of the sleeves are such that when used both individually and in combination, they effectively reproduce the decline in activity of the ^{99m}Tc seen over 96 h (Figure 13.1). The sleeves should be examined carefully prior to use; they will not yield accurate readings if there are any cracks or dents. The initial linearity check should be performed with the slower method of measuring a sample as it decays. Linearity should be checked at *installation* of the device, *quarterly*, and *after repairs* or *when the instrument is moved* to a new location within the clinic.

Geometry

The apparent activity of a dose will vary with the volume and shape of the container and the position of the dose within the chamber. The effect of sample

---

Essentials of Nuclear Medicine Physics and Instrumentation, Third Edition. Rachel A. Powsner, Matthew R. Palmer, and Edward R. Powsner.
© 2013 John Wiley & Sons, Ltd. Published 2013 by John Wiley & Sons, Ltd.

geometry can be tested by placing a small amount of activity at the bottom of a container and progressively adding a diluent such as water. This procedure should be repeated for each type of container used in the laboratory—vials, syringes, bottles, and so on. The left side of Figure 13.2 illustrates photon absorption in a relatively large volume of diluent; the right side illustrates photon loss through the calibrator opening when the sample is placed in a taller container. Dose measurements should not vary by more than 10%. The effect of sample geometry should be checked at *installation* and *after repairs*.

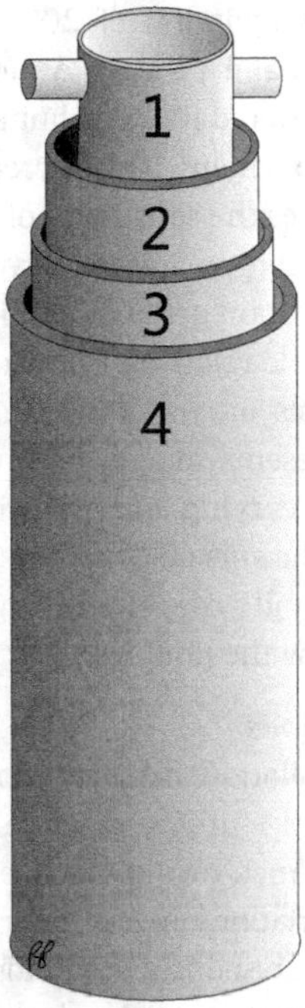

Survey meters

Constancy
A long-lived radioactive source should be checked *daily* to ensure that the meter reading of the source is constant (within 10% of its original value). If the reading differs by more than 10% of the original value, the survey meter should be recalibrated. Typically, the source is attached to the side of the survey meter.

Calibration
All survey meters, including Geiger counters, must be checked for accuracy. To do so, readings are taken from two long-lived sources (^{57}Co and ^{137}Cs) at incremental distances (such as every tenth of a meter up to one meter) from the sources. The sources should be radioactive enough to generate readings at approximately one-third and two-thirds of full scale. The readings must be within 20% of the expected measurement. This test should be performed at *installation, after repairs,* and *annually.*

Figure 13.1 Linearity sleeves.

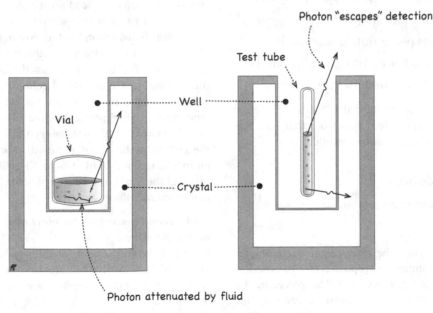

Figure 13.2 Variation in sample geometry.

Crystal scintillation detectors: well counters and thyroid probes

Calibration

On a *daily* basis or prior to each patient measurement, the photopeak is checked using a long-lived nuclide reference source (usually ^{137}Cs), which is placed in the well counter or in front of the probe. The voltage or gain settings are adjusted manually or automatically for the maximum count rate at the peak; the settings and the peak count rate should be recorded. The count rate should not differ from the previous average values or a similarly established value by more than 10%. The full width at half-maximum (FWHM) of the photopeak should be less than 10% of the energy of the photopeak. Calibration should also be routinely performed *annually* and *following repairs*.

Efficiency

This *annual* test is performed using reference standard sources with emissions of similar energy to the nuclides measured routinely in the counter or in front of the thyroid probe. For example, for the thyroid probe, barium-133 (principal gamma emission 356 keV) can be used as a reference for iodine-131 (364 keV), and cobalt-57 (122 keV) can be used for iodine-123 (157 keV).

The **efficiency** of a thyroid probe or well counter can be calculated using the following equation:

Efficiency in cpm/dpm

= [(counts per minute of standard)

− (counts per minute of background)/

(activity of standard in Bq × 60)

This result is often multiplied by 100 and expressed as a percentage value. Remember that one becquerel equals one decay per second.

Imaging devices

Planar gamma camera

Photopeak

Prior to imaging, the pulse-height analyzer may require adjustment to properly center the window of photon energies accepted. The procedure for adjustment differs from camera to camera. One simple procedure for checking the location of the energy window is to place a vial or syringe containing a small quantity of an isotope against the collimator. The computer screen displays a plot of counts vs. energy and the current location of the window (see Figure 5.6). The user can then adjust the location and width of the window. For example, a standard setting for technetium-99m is a photopeak of 140 keV and a window of 20%. The window is set between 126 and 154 keV. A narrower window rejects more scattered photons but also reduces the counts from the patient. This increases the resolution but decreases the sensitivity of the camera.

Drift of the energy window away from the peak will lead to significant artifacts in images. Off-center windows will yield relatively "hot" or "cold" photomultiplier defects on the daily uniformity floods. Figure 13.3 presents images of a uniform source acquired with varying energy windows. In the upper images, the energy window is centered above the photopeak, and in the lower images, the window is centered below the photopeak.

Uniformity floods

Ideally, a scintillation camera should produce a uniform image of a uniform source. Unfortunately, this ideal is not met, owing to imperfections in the collimators, variations in crystal response, differences among the responses of photomultiplier tubes, and minor fluctuations in the electrical circuitry.

The uniformity of the camera's response can be checked by imaging a flood source. A solid plastic disk manufactured with 5–20 mCi of ^{57}Co uniformly distributed throughout its extent, or a fluid-filled sheet source containing a dilute solution of radioactivity, is placed directly on the collimator; this is called an **extrinsic flood field**. Alternatively, a point source is suspended several feet (at a distance three to four times the diameter of the crystal) directly above the surface of the crystal, from which the collimator has been removed; this is called an **intrinsic flood field**. A 5- to 30-million-count image of the flood is then collected according to the manufacturer's directions.

Daily visual inspection for marked nonuniformity

Images of the flood source should be collected and examined *daily*. The human eye can discern variations in counts that are as small as 15%. A uniform flood image is shown in Figure 13.4. If the image does not appear to be uniform, corrective action is

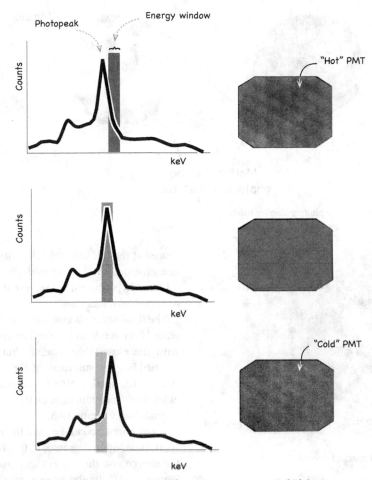

Figure 13.3 Nonuniformity due to off-center energy windows. (Images courtesy of Philip Livingston, CNMT.)

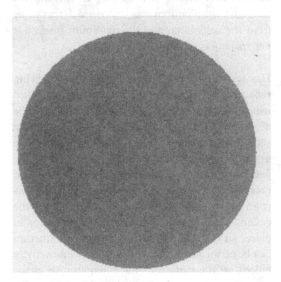

Figure 13.4 Uniform flood field.

required. An example of nonuniformity is shown in Figure 13.5, where a large, rounded defect suggests malfunction of a photomultiplier tube. This corresponds to a similar defect in an image of the thyroid. Less common, but more serious, is the sharply demarcated defect caused by a crack in the crystal (Figure 13.6). These defects are detectable with or without the collimator in place. A subtler example of nonuniformity, from slow drift in the energy window circuitry over a period of three weeks, is shown in Figure 13.7. A damaged collimator can cause linear photopenic defects.

Correction of nonuniformity

In addition to the visual inspection, a flood source collected without collimation (intrinsic) is imaged and loaded into the computer (weekly for older

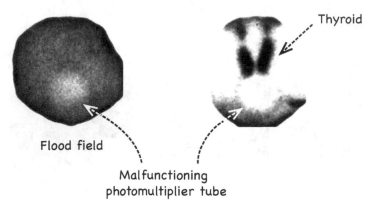

Figure 13.5 Effect of defective photomultiplier tube.

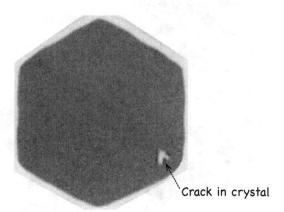

Figure 13.6 Effect of cracked crystal.

camera systems, but much less frequently for newer systems). The computer identifies regions in which counts differ significantly from the mean counts. To compensate for these differences, the computer determines a correction for each pixel, which will later be applied when the camera is used to image a patient. The correction data stored in the computer are referred as the **uniformity correction matrix**. Figure 13.8 is a simplistic representation of the application of a uniformity correction matrix.

Spatial resolution

Bar phantom: The resolution of the imaging system can be evaluated visually by imaging a **bar phantom**. One type of bar phantom is made of lead bars encased in Lucite. The phantom is divided into four quadrants, and the bars in each quadrant are spaced at regular intervals; this interval is different in each quadrant. The intervals illustrated in Figure 13.9 are hypothetical but representative of a standard configuration.

The flood source is imaged with the bar phantom placed between it and the collimator. The quadrant with the closest bar spacing that can be distinguished is a measurement of the resolution of the system. The spatial resolution is checked *weekly* (or at intervals recommended by the manufacturer) for degradation of resolution.

A bar phantom can be used to demonstrate that spatial resolution decreases as the distance between the source and the camera increases, as shown in Figure 13.10. In the images on the left, the bar phantom was placed directly on the collimator; the minimum resolvable bar spacing is 4.0 mm. On the right, the phantom was positioned 10 cm away from the collimator, and the minimum resolvable bar spacing is 4.8 mm.

Line spread function: At installation and following repair, the spatial resolution of the system is checked using the **line spread function**. This can be accomplished by placing a lead mask containing slits (the NEMA line pattern) over the camera face once the collimator has been removed, and suspending a point source several feet above the lead mask to create a series of lines on the crystal. This is an intrinsic test, as it is performed without the collimator on the crystal. With the collimator in place, an extrinsic test of the line spread function can be performed with a line source of radioactivity placed on the surface of the collimator. In either case, the image of the line is broader and less dis-

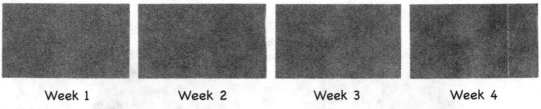

Week 1   Week 2   Week 3   Week 4

Figure 13.7 Nonuniformity due to drift in the circuitry.

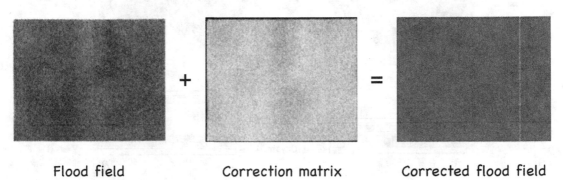

Flood field   Correction matrix   Corrected flood field

Figure 13.8 Uniformity correction matrix.

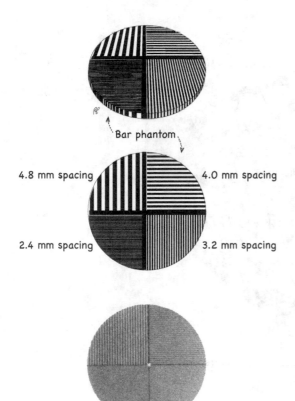

Bar phantom

4.8 mm spacing   4.0 mm spacing

2.4 mm spacing   3.2 mm spacing

Image of bar phantom

Figure 13.9 Bar phantom.

tinct than the slit or line source for a variety of reasons, including acceptance of angled photons, scatter in the material around the source and in the crystal, and imperfections in the camera circuitry (Figure 13.11). Figure 13.12 contains a plot of the distribution of counts in a horizontal slice through the image of the source (the breadth is dependent on the characteristics of the photons and the imaging system). The **full width at half-maximum** (FWHM) and **full width at tenth-maximum** (FWTM) are measurements of the spread of this curve (thus the name "line spread function"). The FWHM is the width of the curve at half the peak count; likewise, the FWTM is the width of the curve at one-tenth of the maximum counts. A system with better resolution will have a narrower curve, and therefore a smaller FWHM and FWTM.

Linearity

The linearity of the gamma camera image is tested by examining the image of a bar phantom obtained with a high-resolution collimator in place. The lines in the image should be straight and unbroken. Note that "linearity" here refers to the appearance of the bars as lines, whereas the same word in reference to the dose calibrator refers to the relationship between dose and meter reading.

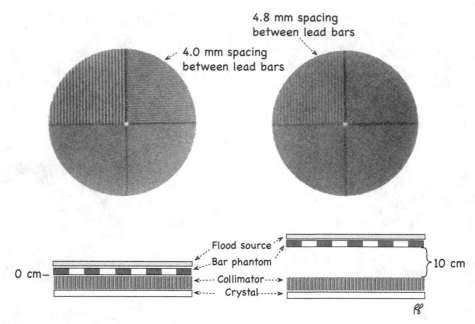

Figure 13.10 Degradation of resolution with distance.

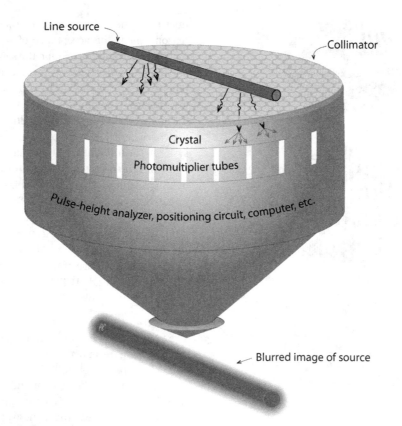

Figure 13.11 Blurring of a line source.

Modulation transfer function

An alternative presentation of these data is achieved by expressing the line spread function in the frequency domain. This is an application of the Fourier transformation described in Chapter 11. As we discussed before, images can be represented as a collection of waves in frequency space. Plots of the **modulation transfer function** show the ability of the camera to reproduce these waves at each spatial frequency. Each camera system has a unique frequency response. This is analogous to stereo systems; some reproduce more of the treble (higher-frequency waves),

others reproduce more of the bass (lower-frequency waves), and the better the system, the more of both bass and treble it can reproduce.

In nuclear medicine systems, the higher frequencies are necessary to reproduce the sharp edges and fine details of an image; the lower and middle frequencies produce the remainder of the image. Figure 13.13 contains plots of the modulation transfer functions of two hypothetical camera systems. System A accepts a greater proportion of lower frequencies, whereas system B accepts a greater proportion of higher frequencies.

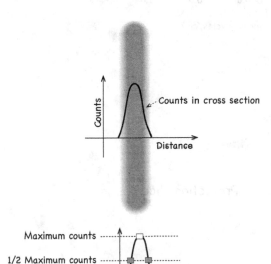

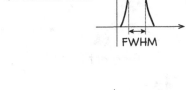

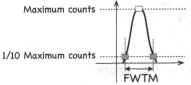

Figure 13.12 Full width at half-maximum and full width at tenth-maximum.

SPECT

The following additional quality control procedures are necessary for SPECT cameras. The frequency of performance of these tests will vary according to the manufacturer's recommendations.

Uniformity

SPECT images are degraded by small degrees of nonuniformity in the flood field that do not adversely affect planar images. It is important to acquire the **flood uniformity correction** for approximately 100 million counts (depending on the manufacturer's recommendations) to reduce nonuniformity caused by statistical variations in count rate. During backprojection, relatively minor defects will become quite prominent and sometimes appear as ring artifacts in the reconstructed transaxial slices. The camera head effectively "drags" the defect with it as it circles the patient. Figure 13.14 illustrates this effect.

Center of rotation

It is assumed that the camera heads will rotate in a near-perfect circle and that the heads will remain almost precisely aligned in their opposing positions. It is also assumed that the predicted, or "electronic," center of the path of rotation will match the "mechanical," or actual, center of the camera head rotation. Deviation from either expectation will degrade image resolution and can be seen as a displacement of the **center of rotation** (COR). Probably the most common cause of apparent displacement of the COR is inadvertent errors (not leveling the camera head, bumping the table,

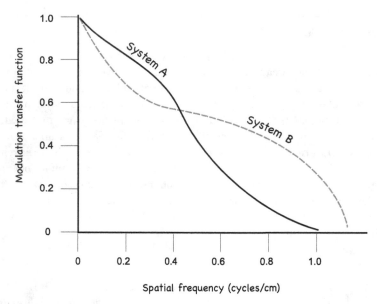

Figure 13.13 Modulation transfer function.

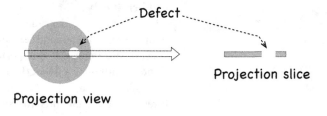

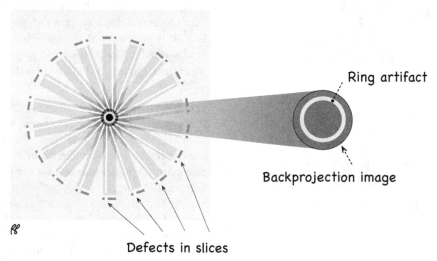

Figure 13.14 Ring artifact created during backprojection of an area of nonuniformity.

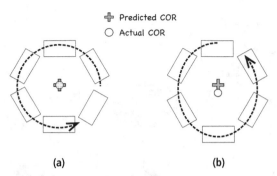

Figure 13.15 Deviation of the mechanical COR.

and so on) during data collection. The most common cause of true shifts of the COR is electronic malfunction. Mechanical problems, such as the use of a collimator that is too heavy for the gantry, are less common. Figure 13.15(a) illustrates a near-perfect circular rotation path for a camera. The predicted COR (cross) is aligned with the actual (mechanical) COR (circle). Figure 13.15(b) illustrates an "unintended" elliptical orbit caused by a heavy camera head that at the bottom of its orbit drifts downward under the influence of gravity. The center of this elliptical orbit (again shown by a circle) is offset from the center of the predicted circular orbit (cross).

Measurement of COR: The test for center of rotation varies by manufacturer but, in general, a simple scheme consists of placing a point source on the patient bed, on center or off center (depending on the manufacturer) . Projection views are obtained over a 360° arc (upper panel of Figure 13.16). COR tests for dual-headed cameras should be performed for each of the head configurations used for imaging, such as the 90° configuration used for cardiac imaging and the 180° configuration used for whole body SPECT.

There are several ways to analyze the difference between the actual and the predicted COR. One common approach is to plot the position of the point source as a function of camera head position along the circle of rotation and compare this with the predicted values. The location of the point source is plotted in the x (perpendicular to the long axis of the bed) and y (parallel to the long axis of the bed) directions. The position of the source plotted in the x direction should closely approximate a sine wave (lower panel of Figure 13.16). The plot of the image of the source in the y direction (not depicted) should be a straight line. A plot of the

source on a camera with a normal COR is illustrated in the upper portion of Figure 13.17. The bottom graph plots the same source on a camera with the elliptical orbit depicted in Figure 13.15. This plot deviates by several pixels from the expected sine wave (dashed lines). Along a portion of the rotation, the measured position differs by several pixels from the expected position of the source. This COR test is abnormal. Deviations of greater than half of one pixel from the expected position of the source are considered abnormal and should be checked with a second collection. A persistent abnormality will require repair prior to collection of further SPECT studies. The results of the COR calculation are stored in the computer and used to correct subsequent SPECT scans.

Measuring SPECT resolution

Phantoms are fillable objects that are used to assess camera resolution. A phantom can be as simple as a plastic bag or as complex as a model of a slice of the brain. SPECT phantoms are cylindrical Lucite containers in which different-sized rods, cylinders, and/or cones of Lucite are interspersed. The container is then filled with water containing a small amount of radioactivity. Tomographic images of the phantom are collected and the reconstructed slices are inspected for visibility of the Lucite objects. The images should be compared with prior acquisitions for evidence of any degradation in resolution.

PET

The quality control protocols for PET cameras can be quite extensive and vary among manufacturers. Some examples of routine procedures are summarized briefly in this section as an introduction to this topic for the reader.

Energy test

Using a standard source, such as ^{24}Na or ^{68}Ge, the energy peak and window are checked daily for accuracy.

Daily quality control

A common *daily* quality control procedure is the acquisition and evaluation of a scan using an internal source or a separate low-activity source.

For scanners with internal rotating sources such as ^{68}Ge, a **transmission scan** is obtained without the patient in the gantry. Because there is no patient

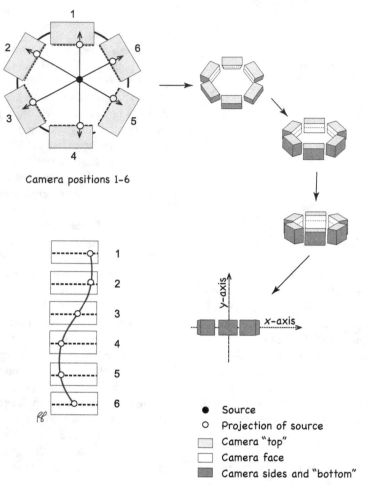

Figure 13.16 COR curves in the *x* direction.

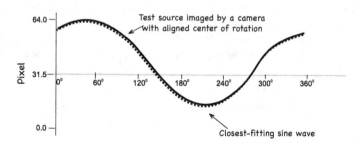

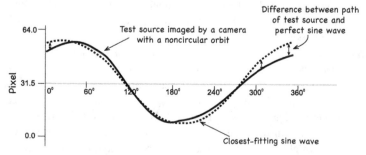

Figure 13.17 Normal and abnormal COR tests.

present, this is sometimes called a **blank scan**. The blank scan is examined for evidence of defective detectors. The data acquired from the blank scan can be displayed as a sinogram. In Chapter 7, we saw that the sinogram (Figure 7.10) was a different way to look at acquired projection views. The sinogram is used in a very similar manner to display PET data. A simplified illustration of the layout of the matrix of detector pairs used to create a PET sinogram for an imaginary camera with 12 detectors is seen in Figure 13.18. Each row of the sinogram contains the counts for all of the opposing detector pairs that have parallel lines of response (the paths between the detectors).

The matrix elements associated with a single detector in this simple system are highlighted in gray and create a diagonal line in Figure 13.19. A normal blank sinogram from a ring detector is

shown in Figure 13.20(a). A defective detector appears as a new thin diagonal line across the sinogram (illustrated in Figure 13.20(b)).

For scanners without internal sources, an **emission scan** is obtained using a source such as a ^{24}Na source placed in the center of the gantry. The data is reconstructed and displayed as a sinogram (Figure 13.21), which has a very different appearance from that seen in the preceding example. This image is examined for discontinuities and deviations from a linear appearance.

During the transmission and emission testing described above, the PMT gains are adjusted. This is possible because the light output from each crystal is predictable when a known quantity of a positron emitter such as ^{68}Ge or ^{24}Na is used. The magnification of a signal from a few electrons to millions of electrons, or the signal gain, that occurs in a

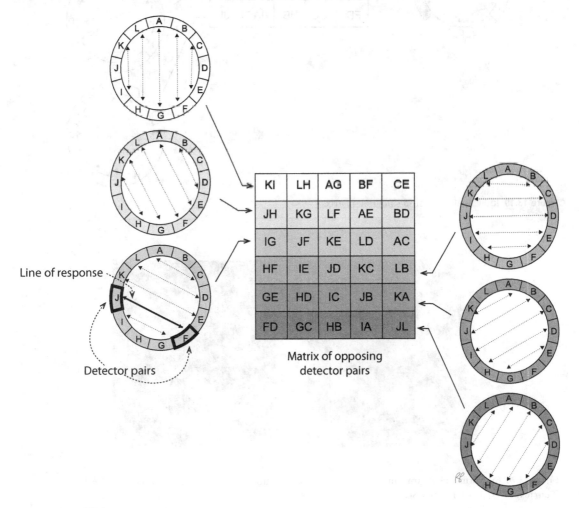

Figure 13.18 PET sinogram matrix.

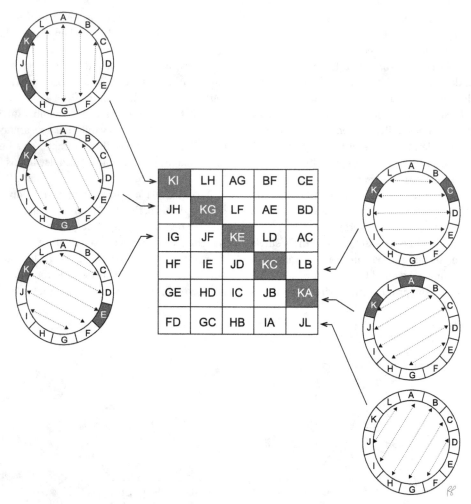

Figure 13.19 Individual detector in sinogram matrix.

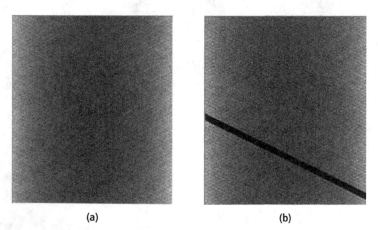

Figure 13.20 (a) Normal blank transmission sinogram. (b) Blank transmission sinogram with a defective detector. (Courtesy of Frederick Fahey, DSc.)

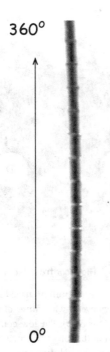

360°

0°

Figure 13.21 Normal emission sinogram.

photomultiplier tube when light photons strike the photocathode end should also be reproducible (see Figure 5.5 and associated text). However, largely as a result of temperature and humidity changes, the PMT response can vary over time. The output from each PMT is measured and adjusted to ensure uniform PMT response.

SUV validation

This *twice-monthly* or *monthly* procedure is used to check the accuracy of the SUV numbers. A small amount of carefully measured positron emitter is diluted in a standard water-filled phantom. The measured activity and time of calibration, as well as the weight and length of the phantom, are entered into the computer. After acquisition and processing, a region of interest is drawn in an attenuation-corrected slice and the calculated SUV value is compared with the expected value. Significant differences indicate a need for recalibration.

Timing resolution test

For PET-CT scanners that utilize time-of-flight circuitry to approximate the location of annihilation events, the time delay between event detection in paired opposing detectors is measured and compared with expected values.

CT

As with PET, CT quality control procedures vary among manufacturers. Although a comprehensive discussion of CT quality control is beyond the scope of this text, a brief introduction to some of the more common procedures is included below.

Tube conditioning

Daily quality control begins with a period of tube conditioning, during which the X-ray tube is gradually warmed up by applying stepwise increments of the kVp. This gradual acclimation prevents tube cracking and electrical arcing.

Air calibration

Daily scanning without a phantom in place is called air calibration, and this is performed with varying combinations of kVp and mAs to adjust the gain of the detectors so that the output or response to the X-ray flux is uniform among the detectors. The resulting images are inspected for artifacts, as are the phantom images discussed next.

CT phantoms

Although individual phantoms could be used to perform each of the following quality control procedures, most CT phantoms are composed of multiple smaller phantoms, and different portions are used for different tests.

CT number quality control

CT number for water, calculation of noise, and visual inspection: A water-filled phantom or a phantom composed of a plastic with a density similar to that of water is scanned, and a large central region of interest is drawn on an image slice. The mean CT number (in Hounsfield units) for the region should be at, or near, the expected CT number of the material: for water, the value is 0, and for plastics the value will be specified by the manufacturer. The standard deviation of the CT number for the region is a measure of the signal **noise** in the image and should be compared with the manufacturer's specifications. An example of a region of interest used for calculating the CT number and standard deviation is depicted by a dashed white circle in Figure 13.22. The image of the phantom is visually inspected for artifacts.

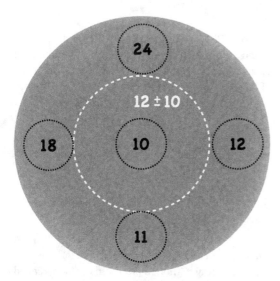

Figure 13.22 Regions of interest used to calculate CT number uniformity and noise. The phantom used for this example was made of plastic.

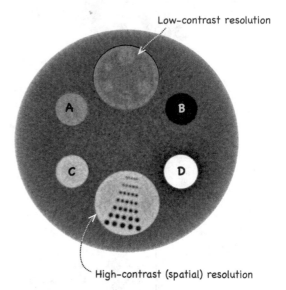

Figure 13.23 Slice of a phantom used to determine CT number accuracy over a wide range of materials (depicted by regions A–D). The low-contrast resolution phantom is seen at the top of the image and the high-contrast spatial-resolution phantom at the bottom.

CT number uniformity: Uniformity of the CT number across the slice is measured by comparing central and peripheral CT numbers within the phantom; these should be within a close range of each other per the manufacturer's specifications. Sample central and peripheral regions of interest are delineated by dashed black lines in Figure 13.22.

CT number linearity: A separate phantom or a portion of a larger phantom, containing materials of different densities, such as Teflon, nylon, and water, is scanned to ascertain the accuracy of CT numbers over a wider range of numbers similar to those encountered in scanning the human body. The images of four regions composed of materials of different densities are labeled A–D in Figure 13.23.

Low-contrast resolution
A phantom containing objects of steadily decreasing size made of materials with similar CT numbers to the background (such as polystyrene cylinders in water or water-filled holes in a polystyrene background) is used to evaluate the resolution when there is little contrast between an object and the background. This phantom simulates the small differences in contrast between the different types of soft tissue found in the human body. An example of an image of a low-contrast resolution phantom can be seen at the top of Figure 13.23.

Spatial (high-contrast) resolution
Spatial resolution can be tested using a phantom somewhat similar to the bar phantom used in SPECT imaging. Phantoms for this purpose are composed of patterns of alternating equally sized pieces of materials. The pattern is repeated with elements of steadily decreasing size. Unlike the low-contrast phantom, the materials have significantly different densities, such as holes or lines (containing air) cut into an aluminum or acrylic glass disk. The phantom is scanned, and the image is examined for the smallest resolvable pattern. An example of this type of phantom can be seen at the bottom of Figure 13.23.

Hybrid system testing
Intermittently, SPECT-CT and PET-CT scanners are checked for accuracy of registration of the PET and CT or SPECT and CT images. One method uses a framework containing several sets of paired radionuclide and radiopaque sources fixed to the pallet. This construct is sequentially scanned using the CT and SPECT or PET components. The reconstructed PET and CT or SPECT and CT images are then visually inspected to ascertain that the paired sources overlap (i.e., are aligned).

Questions

1. Match each of the following quality control procedures with the recommended frequency of performance:
   (a) Dose calibrator linearity.
   (b) Dose calibrator constancy.
   (c) Survey meter constancy.
   (d) Dose calibrator geometry.
   (e) Well counter efficiency.
      (1) Daily.
      (2) Quarterly.
      (3) Annually.
      (4) At installation, after repairs, and when equipment is moved.

2. True or false: A 5-million-count daily uniformity flood can be used to create the uniformity correction matrix for SPECT imaging.

3. Which of the listed quality control procedures might detect the following camera problems (more than one answer per question is possible)?
   Camera problem:
   (a) Drift of the energy window.
   (b) Malfunction of a photomultiplier tube.
   (c) Collimator damage.
   (d) Decrease in spatial resolution.

   Quality control procedure:
   (1) Extrinsic flood.
   (2) Intrinsic flood.
   (3) Flood source with bar phantom.
   (4) Checking the photopeak.

4. True or false: In assessing the results of a center-of-rotation test, a deviation of the measured position of the source of less than two pixels from the expected position does not need further investigation.

5. Match the following quality control procedures with the imaging system:
   Quality control procedure:
   (a) SUV validation.
   (b) Tube conditioning.
   (c) Air calibration.
   (d) Timing resolution test.
   (e) Center-of-rotation test.

Imaging system:
(1) PET.
(2) CT.
(3) SPECT.

6. True or false: Tube conditioning is performed at the start of CT quality control to warm up the X-ray tube and thereby prevent tube cracking or electrical arcing.

7. Which two of the following procedures are used to test dose calibrator linearity?
   (a) A long-lived radioactive source such ^{137}Cs is placed in the dose calibrator and is measured at each energy setting to make sure the response is linear from day to day.
   (b) A vial containing 200 mCi of ^{99m}Tc pertechnetate is placed in the dose calibrator and measured at regular intervals for several days to make sure the readings match the predicted decay values for the sample.
   (c) A vial containing 200 mCi of ^{99m}Tc pertechnetate is placed within lead sleeves of different thickness, which are then combined such that the overall thickness of the lead reproduces the decline in activity of the source over time.

8. Match the name of the CT quality control test with the composition of the phantom:
   (a) Low-contrast resolution.
   (b) Spatial (high-contrast) resolution.
      (1) Objects of decreasing size made of a material with a similar density to the background material, used to simulate the small differences in densities of soft tissues.
      (2) Patterns of two alternating materials of steadily decreasing size. The two materials are of markedly different densities.

9. Calculate the efficiency of a well counter for cobalt-57 given the following information: The reading for a 500 Bq source is 25,000 cpm and the background reading is 200 cpm.

Answers

1. (a) (2). (b) (1). (c) (1). (d) (4). (e) (3).
2. False: A high-count flood, of approximately 100 million counts, is necessary for SPECT uniformity correction.
3. (a) (4), (1), and (2). (b) (1) or (2). (c) (1) or (3). (d) (3).
4. False: Deviations greater than half of one pixel are abnormal and should be checked with a second collection. A persistent abnormality will require repair prior to further SPECT studies.
5. (a) (1). (b) (2). (c) (2). (d) (1). (e) (3).
6. True.
7. (b) and (c). Choice (a) is a description of the dose calibrator constancy test.
8. (a) (1). (b) (2).
9. $(25,000 - 200)$ counts/min/(500 decays/s $\times\ 60$ s/min) = $24,800/30,000$ cpm/dpm = 0.83 cpm/dpm, or 83%.

CHAPTER 14

Radiation Biology

The biological effect of radiation can be understood in terms of the transfer of energy from radiation (photons and particles) to tissue. When the energy of radiation is deposited in the body, it can disrupt chemical bonds and alter tissue. It is important to understand some of the details of this transfer. The interaction of radiation and tissue is governed by the energy and mass of the incident radiation (alpha particles, beta particles, gamma rays, or X-rays) and the properties of the tissue.

Radiation units

Radiation Absorbed Dose (rad)

The radiation absorbed dose, or **rad**, is a measure of the energy transferred to any material from ionizing radiation. The corresponding Système International (SI) unit is the **gray** (Gy), named after the English physicist Louis Harold Gray. Remember that "ionizing radiation" is a term that applies to any radiation that is sufficiently energetic to create ion pairs; it includes X-rays, gamma rays, alpha and beta particles, and neutrons and protons. One gray is equal to 1 joule of energy absorbed per kilogram of tissue; one gray is equal to 100 rad. For example, a bladder wall receives approximately 0.04 Gy (4 rad) from its contained urine following the excretion of a 740 MBq (20 mCi) intravenous dose of ^{99m}Tc-pertechnetate.

Roentgen equivalent man (rem)

The roentgen equivalent man, or **rem**, is the unit of absorbed energy that takes into account the estimated biological effect of the type of radiation that imparts the energy to the tissue. Particles with higher linear energy transfer (LET), such as alpha particles, protons, and neutrons, produce greater tissue damage per rad than do beta particles, gamma rays, or X-rays. The relative damage for each type of radiation is referred to as its **radiation weighting factor** (W_R), values for which are given in Table 14.1.

The **dose equivalent** (or **absorbed energy**) is represented by the letter H (or H_T) and is the product of the dose and the radiation weighting factor, or

H = dose equivalent (in rem)

$\quad$ ▪ absorbed dose (in rad) $\times W_R$

In SI units, we have

H = dose equivalent (in sieverts)

$\quad$ = absorbed dose (in Gy) $\times W_R$

The quantities and units used to measure radiation in nuclear medicine are given in Table 14.2.

The effects of radiation on living organisms

The effects of radiation on living organisms can be described at the level of the cell, a tissue, an entire organism, or a whole population.

Cellular effects

Individual cells

Cellular structure: Cells are the building blocks of living matter and are composed of a nucleus and

Essentials of Nuclear Medicine Physics and Instrumentation, Third Edition. Rachel A. Powsner, Matthew R. Palmer, and Edward R. Powsner.

cytoplasm. The nucleus contains the genetically important chromosomes, which are composed of **deoxyribonucleic acid** (DNA), a large molecule consisting of thousands of small subunits (nucleotides) coiled into a double helix. Each nucleotide is composed of a sugar, a phosphate group, and a base. The genetic code for the cell and for the entire organism is held in the sequence of pairs of bases along the two strands of the double helix. During the process of cell division, called **mitosis**, the DNA reproduces itself so that a complete set of chromosomes is deposited within each cell. In this way, the genetic code is propagated. Since DNA plays such a pivotal role in cellular multiplication and function, radiation damage to DNA has a profound impact on living tissue. Chromosomes are particularly radiosensitive (vulnerable to radiation damage) during mitosis.

Table 14.1 Radiation weighting factors (W_R) for ionizing radiation

Ionizing radiation	W_R
Alpha	20
Neutrons	Varies with neutron energy
Protons	2
Beta (electrons and positrons)	1
Gamma and X-rays	1

Source: ICRP, 2003. Relative Biological Effectiveness (RBE), Quality Factor (Q), and Radiation Weighting Factor (WR). ICRP Publication 92. Ann. ICRP 33(4). (Adapted from Table 1.2: Radiation weighting factors, p. 11)

DNA contains two chains of alternating sugar molecules and phosphate groups. The sugars of the chains are linked by pairs of **bases**—thymine, cytosine, adenine, or guanine. The term "base" refers to the basic, as opposed to acidic, nature of the isolated compounds. These four bases are commonly referred to by their initial letters—T, C, A, and G. The chains and bases are arranged in two long, coiled, intertwined strands, which are tightly packed to form a **chromatid** (Figure 14.1). Two identical chromatids are "attached" to a centromere and form a **chromosome**. As shown at the bottom of Figure 14.1, the bases form pairs across the strands as follows: adenine pairs with thymine, and guanine with cytosine.

The human cell contains 23 pairs of chromosomes; one member of each matched pair is inherited from one of the individual's parents, and the other member from the other parent. One of the pairs of chromosomes determines the individual's sex; male children inherit an X chromosome from their mother and a Y chromosome from their father, and female children inherit an X chromosome from each of their parents. The long strand of DNA within each chromosome contains thousands of genes, each of which contains information from which the cell can manufacture specific proteins.

Mechanisms of radiation damage to DNA: Ionizing radiation can cause deletions or substitutions of bases and/or breaks in the DNA chain. Ionizing particles (neutrons, alpha particles, and beta particles) cause biological damage. Photons (X-rays and gamma rays) transfer energy to "fast" electrons (via Compton

Table 14.2 Quantities and units used in nuclear medicine

Quantity	Système International (SI) unit	Conventional unit	Equivalence	Meaning
Activity (A)	becquerel (Bq)	curie (Ci)	$1\,Bq = 2.7 \times 10^{-11}\,Ci$	Number of disintegrations of radioactive material per second
Absorbed dose (D)	gray (Gy)	rad	$1\,Gy = 100\,rad$	Energy absorbed from ionizing radiation per unit mass of absorber
Exposure	coulombs per kilogram (C/kg)	roentgen (R)	$1\,C/kg = 3.9 \times 10^3\,R$	Amount of charge liberated by ionizing radiation per unit mass of air
Dose equivalent (H)	sievert (Sv)	rem	$1\,Sv = 100\,rem$	Absorbed dose times the radiation weighting factor (dose $\times W_R$)

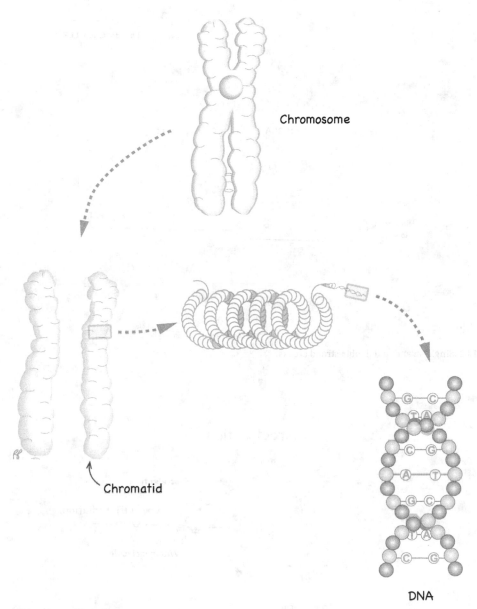

Figure 14.1 The structure of chromosomes and DNA.

scattering and the photoelectric effect), which in turn cause biological damage through ionization.

Base deletions or substitutions can have variable effects on the cell line. DNA strand breaks, if not repaired, cause abnormalities in chromosomes that may result in cell death. **Single breaks**, caused by low-LET (see Chapter 3) radiation given at a low dose rate, are relatively easily repaired by using the other strand of DNA as a template. Radiation of relatively high LET, or a high dose rate of low-LET radiation, may produce single breaks in close prox-

imity to each other in both strands (called **double- or multiple-strand breaks**), which are more difficult to repair (Figure 14.2).

Direct and indirect action of radiation: DNA damage can occur as a result of **direct action**, in which particulate radiation (such as alpha particles) or fast electrons produced by photons in Compton and photoelectron interactions strike the DNA molecules (Figure 14.3). Alternatively, damage may be caused by **indirect action**, in which the radiation

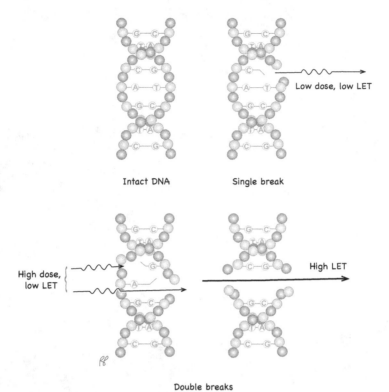

Intact DNA   Single break

Low dose, low LET

High dose,
low LET

High LET

Double breaks

Figure 14.2 Single-strand and double-strand breaks.

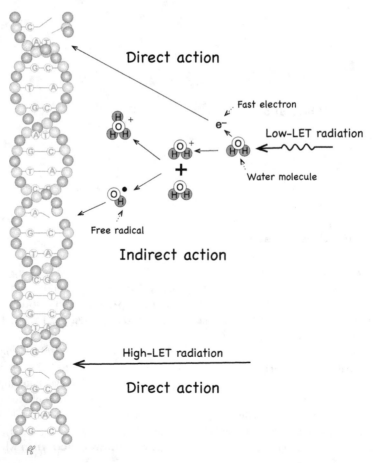

Direct action

Fast electron

e⁻

Low-LET radiation

Water molecule

Free radical

+

Indirect action

High-LET radiation

Direct action

Figure 14.3 Direct and indirect action.

interacts with water molecules in the cell to form free radicals (see box), which in turn damage the DNA strands (see Figure 14.3 again). Most DNA damage caused by low-LET radiation is a result of indirect action. Most DNA damage caused by high-LET radiation is via direct action.

Free radicals

Indirect DNA damage is mediated by free radicals. When particulate or photon radiation interacts with water (H_2O), an ion pair (H_2O^+, e^-) is formed. The electron combines with an H_2O molecule to form H_2O^-. The H_2O^+ and H_2O^- are called ion radicals (not to be confused with free radicals). Ion radicals are very unstable and rapidly dissociate: H_2O^+ becomes H^+ and $OH^\cdot$, and H_2O^- becomes $H^\cdot$ and OH^-. $OH^\cdot$ and $H^\cdot$ are free radicals.

A free radical is an atom or molecule that has no electrical charge, but is highly reactive because it has an odd number of electrons with an unpaired electron in its outer shell. Free radicals tend to quickly recombine to form stable electron configurations. However, in high enough concentrations in the cell, they can create organic free radicals ($R^\cdot$) and H_2O_2 (hydrogen peroxide), a toxic molecule. $OH^\cdot$ + RH become $R^\cdot$ + H_2O, and two $OH^\cdot$ become H_2O_2. Organic free radicals in DNA lead to breakage of the strands and crosslinking. $OH^\cdot$, since it oxidizes (removes electrons), is more damaging than $H^\cdot$, which is a reducing agent (gives up its electrons).

Radiosensitivity and cell cycle: The normal mitotic cycle of the cell is illustrated in Figure 14.4. The **cell cycle** can be divided into four segments, the lengths of which vary as a function of the cell type. During **mitosis**, the cell divides into two individual cells. This is followed by **interphase G_1**, during which only one copy of the cellular DNA is contained in a chromatid. The **synthetic (S) phase** is a period of DNA replication. In **interphase G_2**, the chromatid has duplicated, and the DNA is doubled and is located in chromosomes.

Experiments have shown that the cell is relatively resistant to radiation damage during the latter part of the S phase, the period of DNA synthesis. It is hypothesized that during this portion of the cell cycle, the relative abundance of repair enzymes (DNA polymerase and ligase) facilitates DNA repair. Other experiments have shown that the greatest amount of damage occurs during the period of mitosis; the dose needed to halt mitotic activity in a dividing cell is much less than that needed to destroy the function of a differentiated cell. The latter portion of the G_2 phase is nearly as sensitive as the mitotic phase.

Cell survival curves

Thus far, we have outlined the effects of radiation on individual cells. Since it is likely that cells will be randomly damaged, it is more useful to consider the overall effects of radiation on groups of cells.

The effect of radiation on cell populations is often expressed as a semilogarithmic plot of the fraction of surviving cells versus radiation dose. The surviving cell fraction is plotted along the y-axis using a logarithmic scale and the radiation dose on a linear scale along the x-axis (see Figure 14.5). The actual biophysical mechanisms underlying the observed cell survival curves are felt to be complex and are not fully understood. However, the following explanations for the curve shape, although simplistic, are useful.

Cell survival as a function of radiation dose is exponential (appearing as a straight line on the semilogarithmic plot) for high-LET radiation (bottom plot in Figure 14.5). A likely explanation for this appearance is that most DNA damage with high-LET radiation is via multiple breaks that are generally not repaired. In contrast, cells exposed to lower doses of low-LET radiation can often repair the single-strand breaks caused by this type of radiation. For the lower doses of such radiation, therefore, the fraction of the cells surviving is greater than for a similar dose of high-LET radiation. The initial, relatively more horizontal slope in the low-LET curve likely reflects the cells' ability to repair the single breaks caused during low doses of low-LET radiation (top plot in Figure 14.5). At increasingly higher doses of low-LET radiation, multiple DNA breaks are more likely and the slope of the curve becomes steeper, more closely approximating that for high-LET radiation.

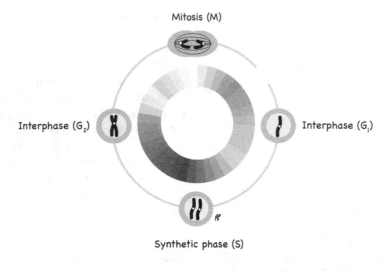

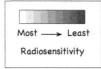

Figure 14.4 The cell cycle and relative radiosensitivity.

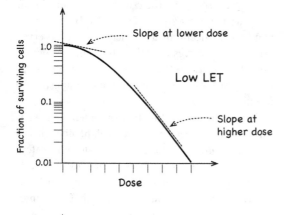

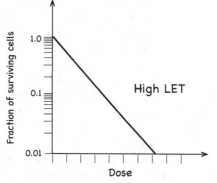

Figure 14.5 Cell survival curves for low- and high-LET radiation.

Factors affecting cell survival

Dose rate

Low-LET radiation: The degree of damage incurred when a dose of low-LET radiation is administered is dependent on the rate at which this dose is delivered. With delivery of a given dose over a longer period of time (lower dose rate), most DNA damage is via single-strand breaks and the cell has time to repair the damage. At high dose rates, there are more multiple-strand breaks and there is less time to repair single-strand breaks. As a result, the initial more horizontal portion of the curve becomes smaller (Figure 14.6).

High-LET radiation: High-LET radiation causes such a high incidence of multiple-strand breaks that repair is negligible at any dose rate.

Chemical interventions: The introduction of certain chemicals into the medium in which the cells exist can alter the cell population's response to administered radiation doses. These chemicals alter the indirect effects (via free radicals) of radiation on DNA.

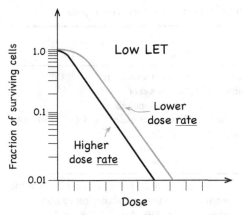

Figure 14.6 Effect of dose rate on cell survival for low-LET radiation.

Radiosensitizers: These substances increase the amount of radiation damage to cells at a given radiation dose and are used in radiation therapy to increase death of tumor cells. Radiosensitizers include oxygen, halogenated pyrimidines, and nitroimidazoles.

• *Oxygen:* Oxygen enhances the indirect action of low-LET radiation by binding to the free radicals R' on damaged ends of DNA breaks. The resulting RO_2' is a more stable free radical, and the damaged ends are less likely to be repaired (Figure 14.7). Oxygen has less effect on the radiotoxicity of high-LET radiation, which is more likely to damage DNA by direct action. The effect of oxygen as a radiosensitizer is most pronounced in anaerobic tissues such as the centers of tumor masses.

The **oxygen enhancement ratio** (OER) is the ratio of the dose in hypoxic tissue to the dose in aerated tissue required to cause a given tissue effect. For photon or X-ray irradiation, this ratio is approximately 2.5 to 3.5 at high doses [1]. For high-LET radiation (alpha particles), the ratio approaches 1.0, since most of the damage is via direct action. Figure 14.8 illustrates an OER of 2.0 from a hypothetical X-ray dose. Half of the X-ray dose is needed during oxygenation to kill the same proportion of the cell population irradiated in anaerobic conditions.

• *Halogenated pyrimidines:* The halogenated pyrimidines 5-iododeoxyuridine and 5-bromodeoxyuridine are very similar to thymine and are easily incorporated in its place into DNA. However, the substitu-

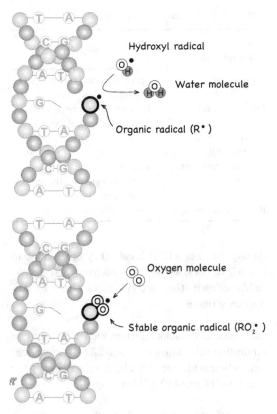

Figure 14.7 Oxygen binds to damaged DNA.

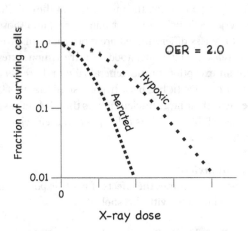

Figure 14.8 Effect of oxygenation on cell survival during low-LET irradiation.

tion "weakens" the DNA, making it more susceptible to radiation damage.

• *Nitroimidazoles:* The nitroimidazoles, including misonidazole and etanidazole, mimic the action of oxygen by binding to the free radical R' on a

Table 14.3 Radiosensitivity of cell types

Relative radiosensitivity	Examples
Highly sensitive	Spermatogonia, erythroblasts, lymphocytes
Relatively sensitive	Epidermal basal cells, intestinal crypt cells, myelocytes
Intermediate sensitivity	Osteoblasts, spermatocytes, chondroblasts
Relatively resistant	Liver cells, spermatozoa, granulocytes, erythrocytes, osteocytes
Highly resistant	Neural cells, muscle cells

Table 14.4 Organ toxicity from acute exposure

Organ	Type of damage	Threshold (Gy (rad))
Ocular lens	Cataract formation	2 (200)[a]
Bone marrow	Depression of hematopoiesis	0.5 (50)
Reproductive organs	Permanent male sterility	3.5–6 (350–600)
	Permanent female sterility	2.5–6 (250–600)

Source: ICRP, 2007. The 2007 Recommendations of the International Commission on Radiological Protection. ICRP Publication 103. Ann. ICRP 37(2-4), p. 164.
[a]There is a latency period for cataract formation of several years ([4], p. 168).

damaged end of a DNA break. They are effective in hypoxic tumors, as they can penetrate more deeply; unlike oxygen, they are not metabolized by surrounding tissue.

Radioprotectors: Radioprotectors, such as cysteine and amifostine (also known as WR-2721), "scavenge" or combine with free radicals, thereby reducing the likelihood of low-LET DNA damage.

Tissue effects

The radiosensitivity of different types of tissues is largely dependent on the mitotic rate of the cells. In general, cells with a higher mitotic rate and those that are less differentiated are more radiosensitive. For reasons not understood, mature lymphocytes are an exception to the general rule and are very radiosensitive (it has been hypothesized that this is because their large nucleus makes the DNA an easy target). Table 14.3 lists cell types and their relative radiosensitivity.

Organ toxicity

Table 14.4 outlines the effects of acute exposure on selected organs, with threshold doses.

Embryo and fetus: Prior to and during early implantation of the embryo, when the cells are pluripotential, it is generally accepted that the embryo will either succumb to radiation or survive without significant abnormalities. Some work suggests that rodent embryos with certain genetic predispositions may survive radiation with malformations that are not lethal [2]. After the time of implantation and during the time of rapid organ development (orga-

nogenesis), organ malformation may occur. Most observed organ damage from radiation during human embryonic and fetal development involves the brain. Table 14.5 outlines the effects of radiation during formation of the embryo and fetus.

Acute whole-body radiation toxicity: Radiosensitivity varies between species. It is expressed as the lethal dose that will kill half of the individuals in a population within 30 days, denoted by **LD$_{50/30}$**. For mice, LD$_{50/30}$ is equal to 5.5 Gy [3]. Human lethal doses are expressed over 60 day intervals. The LD$_{50/60}$ for humans is between 3 and 5 Gy [4]. Acute radiation sickness following whole-body irradiation is discussed in Chapter 17.

Heritable and cancer effects

The adverse effects of radiation exposure include death, tissue damage, the development of cancer, and inherited genetic effects. The risk of developing an adverse effect may be classified as either stochastic or nonstochastic.

Stochastic and nonstochastic risks

Cancer and the genetic effects of radiation are examples of **stochastic risks**. A stochastic risk is the *probability* that exposure to radiation will result in damage to an exposed organism. The likelihood than an individual will develop cancer or suffer from their parents' gonadal exposure to radiation is dose-dependent; the greater the dose, the more likely the adverse effect. However, these likelihoods

Table 14.5 Radiosensitivity of the human embryo and fetus up to week 25

Stage	Characteristics	Time period	Effect
Preimplantation and implantation	Implantation begins on day 6	Days 0–14	"All or nothing": termination or survival without apparent defects[a]
Embryogenesis (organogenesis)	Most major organ systems are formed	Weeks 3–8	Potentially severe organ abnormalities, including growth retardation[a]
Fetal stage	Rapid development of nervous system with increased mitotic activity, neuronal cell proliferation	Weeks 8–15	Highest risk of severe mental retardation, with threshold dose 0.55 Gy.[b] IQ decreases by 25 points/Gy.[c]
	Neuronal cell differentiation and formation of synapses	Weeks 16–25	Continued risk of severe mental retardation, with threshold dose of 0.87 Gy.[b] IQ decreases by 13 points/Gy.[c]

[a]Data based on research on rodents.
[b]ICRP, 2003. Biological Effects after Prenatal Irridation (Embryo and Fetus). ICRP Publication 90. Ann. ICRP 33(1-2). p 106.
[c]ICRP, 2003. Biological Effects after Prenatal Irridation (Embryo and Fetus). ICRP Publication 90. Ann. ICRP 33(1-2). p 108.

are only statistical probabilities; within a population exposed to radiation, it is not known which particular individuals will develop cancer or a genetic defect (unless of course the dose is high enough to create a 100% risk). On the other hand, dose-related risks, also known as **nonstochastic** or **deterministic** risks, do not result from exposure alone, but from **dose-related** exposures. In the latter case, there are thresholds above which radiation damage can be expected in all exposed individuals; for example, receipt of 6 Gy (600 rad) to the eyes will result in the future development of cataracts. The risk is said to be 100% above a threshold of 2 Gy (200 rad).

Heritable effects

The estimated spontaneous or baseline genetic mutation rate is approximately 3×10^{-6} mutations per gene per generation. The **doubling dose** is the dose of low-LET, low-dose radiation that will induce, or cause, a number of genetic mutations equivalent to the baseline rate, and this dose is estimated at 1 Gy.

For such diseases as retinoblastoma and Huntington's chorea, a single mutation in a gene inherited from one parent will cause disease, even in the presence of normal DNA in the comparable gene of the other parent. Inheritance through a single gene constitutes **autosomal dominance**. Similarly, a male child can inherit a genetic mutation on the X

chromosome acquired from his mother where there is no matching gene on the Y chromosome inherited from his father. The resulting conditions are called **X-linked** diseases. The combined baseline incidence for autosomal dominant and X-linked diseases is approximately 16,500 per million births. An additional 750–1500 children with such diseases are born to parents who have been exposed to radiation for each gray of exposure [5]. Therefore the increased incidence per gray of radiation for these inherited diseases is approximately 6%.

There are, however, many inherited chronic diseases, such as diabetes, that occur as a result of more than one genetic mutation combined with environmental factors and, as such, are called **multifactorial diseases**. The natural or baseline risk of manifesting any heritable disease, including these chronic diseases, is high, at 738,000 per million live births. The increased incidence per million children per gray of radiation to their parents for any heritable disease is approximately 4000 cases, or 0.5% of the baseline rate [5].

Carcinogenic effects

The incidence of certain cancers—such as leukemia, and head and neck, pharyngeal, thyroid, breast, and lung cancers—has historically been shown to be increased following radiation exposure. Cancer induction following radiation disasters such as the bombing of Hiroshima and nuclear accidents, and following some medical procedures, has been studied in an attempt to model and quantify risk. Because the data are fairly limited and the natural rate of cancer is so high (there is approximately a 45% lifetime risk of developing cancer), it has been very difficult to determine this risk precisely and, over the years, this has led to a great deal of disagreement and controversy.

Most recently, the BEIR VII committee of the National Academy of Sciences of the USA examined all the available data and considered all leading hypotheses and models, and they concluded that the risk of developing cancer following exposure to low levels of radiation (<100 mSv) is linear with dose and that there is no threshold effect. This is referred as the **linear no-threshold (LNT) hypothesis**—no threshold, because the risk is assumed to be extrapolated down to the most minute dose and therefore the risk, although proportionately minute (and virtually impossible to measure, given the high background rate of cancer), is never zero. That is, radiation causes cancer and there is no "safe level" of radiation—every incidence of exposure carries a certain risk of producing cancer that is proportional to the dose.

Calculating the risk of cancer induction given the radiation dose is not exactly straightforward. For a given dose, the risk of cancer induction is higher in children, for example, than in adults. The risk of cancer induction in the elderly is lower owing to the relatively long lag time before the onset of disease. And, for reasons that are not entirely explained by increased expected lifespan, the risk of radiation-induced cancer induction for women is higher than that for men. Overall, the BEIR VII study estimates the average risk of developing cancer for the US population to be approximately 1% per 100 mSv (Table 12-13 in [6]).

To put this into context, suppose that a person representative of an average member of the US population were to agree to undergo a CT examination of the pelvis as part of a research study. If the examination involved a dose of 10 mSv, then the risk of that study causing cancer would be 0.1% (1% × 10 mSv/100 mSv) or, to frame it in the context of the overall risk of developing cancer, that person's lifetime risk of developing cancer would be increased from 45% to 45.1% as a consequence of taking part in the study.

For patients, concern over the increased risk of cancer from diagnostic radiology and nuclear medicine tests must be weighed against the risk of delaying diagnosis or "underdiagnosing" disease. Judicious use of testing is always advisable; in addition, more attention is now being given to balancing image resolution against radiation burden.

References

1. Hall EJ, and Giaccia, AJ. *Radiobiology for the Radiologist*, 7th edn. Philadelphia: Wolters Kluwer, 2010, p. 86.
2. ICRP, 2003. Biological Effects after Prenatal Irradiation (Embryo and Fetus). ICRP Publication 90. Ann. ICRP 33(1-2). p. 19.
3. Casarett AP. *Radiation Biology*. Englewood Cliffs, NJ: Prentice Hall, 1968, p. 220.
4. ICRP, 2007. The 2007 Recommendations of the International Commission on Radiological Protection. ICRP Publication 103. Ann. ICRP 37(2-4), p. 165.
5. ICRP, 2007. The 2007 Recommendations of the International Commission on Radiological Protection. ICRP Publication 103. Ann. ICRP 37(2-4), p. 231.
6. National Research Council. *Health Risks from Exposure to Low Levels of Ionizing Radiation: BEIR VII Phase 2*. Washington, DC: National Academies Press, 2006, p. 291.

Questions

1. Which of the following statements are correct for the radionuclides used in nuclear medicine imaging?
   - (a) The dose equivalent is ten times the absorbed dose.
   - (b) The dose equivalent is equal to the absorbed dose.
   - (c) The radiation weighting factor, or relative tissue damage per administered gray of radiation, is larger for high-LET radiation than for low-LET radiation.
   - (d) All of the above.

2. True or false: Single-strand DNA breaks, which are caused by low-dose low-LET radiation, are less likely to be repaired than double- or multiple-strand breaks, which are caused by high-dose low-LET radiation or high-LET radiation.

3. Rank the following phases of the cell cycle from the most radiosensitive to the least radiosensitive:
   - (a) Mitosis.
   - (b) Interphase G_1.
   - (c) Synthetic phase (S).
   - (d) Interphase G_2 (latter part).

4. Which of the following are true?
   - (a) Oxygen enhances DNA damage from high-LET radiation more than it enhances DNA damage from low-LET radiation.
   - (b) The oxygen enhancement ratio for low-LET radiation is 1.
   - (c) The oxygen enhancement ratio for high-LET radiation is 2.5 to 3.5.

   - (d) All of the above.
   - (e) None of the above.

5. Connect the following doses or risk factors with their estimated values:
   - (a) Threshold dose in gray above which there is 100% incidence of cataracts.
   - (b) Doubling dose that will increase the genetic mutation rate to twice the baseline rate.
   - (c) Excess relative risk of cancer induction per sievert of low-dose radiation exposure.

   Dose or risk factor value:
   - (1) 2 Gy (200 rad).
   - (2) 0.1%.
   - (3) 1 Gy (100 rad).

6. Rank the following tissues in order from most radiosensitive to most radioresistant:
   - (a) Lymphocytes.
   - (b) Neural cells.
   - (c) Spermatozoa.
   - (d) Erythrocytes.
   - (e) Intestinal crypt cells.

7. The highest risk of radiation-induced severe mental retardation occurs during which stage of embryonic and fetal development?
   - (a) Preimplantation (weeks 0–2).
   - (b) Embryogenesis (organogenesis) (weeks 3–8).
   - (c) Early fetal development (weeks 8–15).

8. True or false: In general, radiation exposure of the preimplantation embryo will result in either survival without malformation or death.

Answers

1. (b) and (c).
2. False.
3. (a), (d), (b), (c).
4. (e).

5. (a) (1). (b) (3). (c) (2).
6. (a), (e), (c), (d), (b).
7. (c).
8. True.

CHAPTER 15

Radiation Dosimetry

Dosimetry is the calculation of the total absorbed radiation dose to individual organs or the whole body from internal and external radiation exposure. The absorbed doses for diagnostic procedures are relatively small, and therefore dosimetry is approximated using phantoms or standardized computer models of the human body and, in the case of nuclear medicine studies, studies of the distribution of radiopharmaceuticals. Therapeutic procedures involve much greater radiation doses, and individual-specific information, such as measurements of the biodistribution of tracer doses and measurements of organ mass based on imaging procedures, is frequently employed to more accurately estimate individual dosimetry. This chapter will discuss some of the methods of dosimetry and the terms used to represent it for diagnostic nuclear medicine procedures, where doses are largely the result of internal exposure, and computed tomography procedures, which involve external radiation exposure.

Nuclear medicine dosimetry

Internal-dosimetry information is supplied with all radiopharmaceuticals, as shown for ^{18}F- fluorodeoxyglucose in Table 15.1. This table contains individual organ doses and the effective dose; in the following text, we shall briefly explore the derivation of these values.

Physical, biological, and effective half-lives

The calculations for internal dosimetry rely on an understanding of the different types of half-lives used to describe radiopharmaceuticals. The **physical half-life** (T_p or $T_{1/2}$) is the time it takes for half

of the nuclide atoms to become stable (see Chapter 1). The **biological half-life** (T_b) has nothing to do with radioactivity, but rather reflects the half-time for excretion of the material from the organ or whole body. For instance, the biological half-life of ^{99m}Tc-MDP is the time it takes for one-half of this radiopharmaceutical to be filtered and excreted by the kidneys and bladder. The **effective half-life** (T_e) is a measurement that combines the above two values; it is the time required for one-half of the initial radioactivity to disappear from an organ or the body both by excretion and by physical decay. The effective half-life is always shorter than either the physical or the biological half-life and is calculated using the formula

$$\frac{1}{T_e} = \frac{1}{T_b} + \frac{1}{T_p}$$

or

$$T_e = \frac{T_b \times T_p}{T_b + T_p}$$

Table 15.2 lists hypothetical values to demonstrate the relationship between the three types of half-lives. Table 15.3 lists actual values for selected radiopharmaceuticals; note that for many radiopharmaceuticals the biokinetics are relatively complex, with more than one biological half-time for each organ.

Calculation of organ doses

Several systems are available for internal-dosimetry calculations. Three of the more commonly used systems are the ICRP (International Committee for Radiation Protection), RADAR (Radiologic Dose Assessment Resource), and MIRD (Medical Internal

Essentials of Nuclear Medicine Physics and Instrumentation, Third Edition. Rachel A. Powsner, Matthew R. Palmer, and Edward R. Powsner.
© 2013 John Wiley & Sons, Ltd. Published 2013 by John Wiley & Sons, Ltd.

198   Essentials of Nuclear Medicine Physics and Instrumentation

Table 15.1 Part of the estimated dosimetry for ^{18}F-FDG

Tissue	Absorbed dose (mGy/MBq)	Absorbed dose (rad/mCi)
Bladder wall	0.16	0.59
Heart	0.062	0.23
Kidneys	0.021	0.078
Red marrow	0.011	0.041
Effective dose (E)	0.019 mSv/MBq	

Adapted from ICRP, 1998. Radiation Dose to Patients from Radiopharmaceuticals (Addendum to ICRP 53), ICRP Publication 80, Ann. ICRP 28(3)

Table 15.2 Physical, biological, and effective half-lives (hypothetical values)

T_p	T_b	T_e
1000	1	0.999
200	100	67
10	10	5
1	1	0.5
10	20	6.7
1	1000	0.999

Table 15.3 Sample physical, biological, and effective half-lives

Radiopharmaceutical	T_p	T_b	T_e
^{99m}Tc–sulfur colloid	6 h	∞[a]	6 h
^{99m}Tc-DTPA	6 h	1.7 h[b]	1.3 h
^{123}I-MIBG	13.2 h	1.4 days[c]	9.5 h
^{131}I	8 days	80 days[d]	7.3 days

Source: IRCP, 1987. Radiation Dose to Patients from Radiopharmaceuticals. ICRP Publication 53, Ann ICRP 18(1-4).
[a]Sulfur colloid is taken up by reticuloendothelial cells and has very slow elimination from the liver, so the biological half-life of the sulfur colloid is estimated as infinite.
[b]Total body excluding bladder contents.
[c]Adrenals only.
[d]Thyroid only.

Radiation Dose) systems. Although the equations they employ for dosimetry calculations appear, at first glance, to be quite different, the underlying principles and components used in the calculations have much in common. The following is a discussion of one such approach, the MIRD system, which, although one of the older models, is useful for demonstration purposes.

Using the MIRD system, the dose delivered to an organ, $\bar{D}$, can be represented as the product of the total (cumulated) activity within the organ, $\tilde{A}$, and S, a conversion factor based on physiologic characteristics of the administered radionuclide and the organ of interest:

$$\bar{D} = \tilde{A} \times S$$

Description of terms
A_0, the **initial activity**, is the amount of injected activity that is in the organ immediately after injection. $A(t)$ is the activity within the organ as a function of time. The **cumulated activity**, $\tilde{A}$, is the summed total activity within the organ over the entire time the radioactivity remains within the organ. The uppermost plot in Figure 15.1 is a time–activity curve; the activity at time 0 is A_0. The area under the curve, $\tilde{A}$, can be approximated by sequential thin rectangles (second uppermost panel). The cumulated activity can be calculated from the initial activity and the effective half-life T_e of the radiopharmaceutical as follows.

The residence time, τ, is the time over which the organ would receive the same total dose from the amount of initial activity (A_0) were this to remain constant and then fall instantly to zero. If one were to rearrange the thin rectangles in the second panel of Figure 15.1 into a large rectangle of height A_0, the width of this rectangle would be τ (lower panels):

$$\tilde{A} = \tau \times A_0$$

The residence time is related to the effective half-life (discussed above) by the equation

$$\tau = 1.44 \times T_e$$

It then follows that

$$\tilde{A} = 1.44 \times T_e \times A_0$$

S Value: The radiation dose $\bar{D}$ to any organ depends on the activity accumulated in that organ ($\tilde{A}$), on the size, shape, and density of the organ, and on the energy and type of radiation emitted by the activity that it contains; for penetrating radiation, it also depends on the energy and type of radiation emitted by accumulated activity in other organs in the body (this will be covered in the next section). We have already discussed how cumulated activity can be calculated, but the calculation for the remaining factors is too complicated to pursue here. Fortunately,

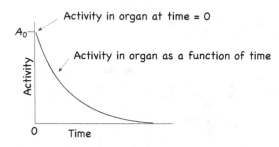

Activity in organ at time = 0

Activity in organ as a function of time

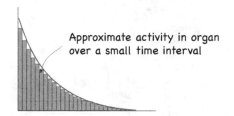

Approximate activity in organ
over a small time interval

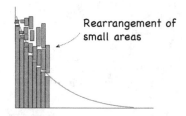

Rearrangement of
small areas

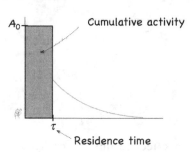

Cumulative activity

Residence time

Figure 15.1 Time–activity curve, cumulated activity, and residence time.

these calculations have been performed for most of the organs of the body and for the range of photon and particle energies emitted by the medically important radionuclides. The resulting combined factors are referred to as the **S values**, which are available in standard tables. For the curious, an in-depth demonstration of the calculation of an S value is presented in Appendix C.

Self-dose, target, and source organs: The term **self-dose** is used to describe the radiation dose to an organ from a radionuclide within it, for example the dose to the liver from the accumulation of ^{99m}Tc–

sulfur colloid in the liver. The same approach can be applied to calculate the dose to any organ of the body, the **target**, from the radioactivity of any other organ, called the **source** (for example, the dose to the thyroid from ^{99m}Tc–sulfur colloid in the liver). The left side of Figure 15.2 depicts the liver as the source organ and all organs, including the liver, as target organs. In the part on the right, the lung is the source organ following injection of ^{99m}Tc-MAA. The total dose to any organ, considered as a target, is the sum of the doses from all sources within the body. There are S values for each combination of source and target organs.

Sample calculation of $\bar{D}$

A sample calculation of an absorbed dose may elucidate the above concepts. We shall use a hypothetical case of ^{131}I sodium iodide ingestion with the lung as the target organ and the thyroid as the source organ. To simplify the calculation, we shall assume that the thyroidal uptake of ^{131}I sodium iodide is instantaneous and that the radioiodine uptake is 30%. The ingested dose is 1 mCi (37 MBq).

The initial activity in the thyroid is

$$A_0 = 1\,\text{mCi} \times 30\%\,\text{uptake}$$
$$= 0.3\,\text{mCi}\,(11.1\,\text{MBq})$$

The effective half-life (see Table 15.2) is

$$T_e = 7\,\text{days}$$

The residence time is

$$\tau = 1.44 \times T_e$$
$$= 10\,\text{days}$$

The cumulated activity is

$$\tilde{A} = \tau \times A_0$$
$$= 10\,\text{days} \times 0.3\,\text{mCi}$$
$$= 3\,\text{mCi days}$$
$$= 72\,\text{mCi h}\,(2664\,\text{MBq h})$$

The S value when the source is the thyroid and the target is the lung is calculated as 2.9×10^{-6} rad/µCi h [1]. The absorbed dose to the lungs from the thyroid is

$$\bar{D} = \tilde{A} \times S$$
$$= 72{,}000\,\mu\text{Ci h} \times 2.9 \times 10^{-6}\,\text{rad/}\mu\text{Ci h}$$
$$= 0.21\,\text{rad}\,(0.0021\,\text{Gy})$$

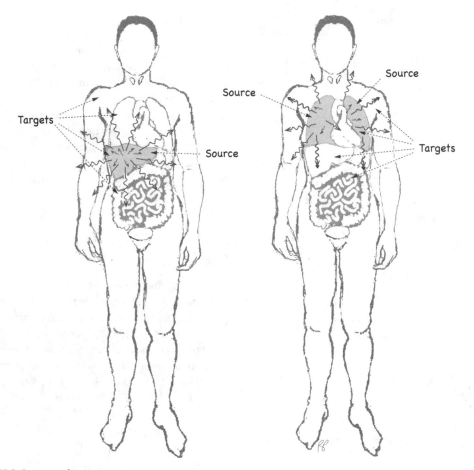

Figure 15.2 Source and target organs.

Effective dose

A value called the **total body dose**, sometimes published in dosimetry tables for radiopharmaceuticals, is calculated as the total energy deposited in the body divided by an average body mass. This calculation, however, does not factor in the relative radiosensitivity of organs in terms of the relative risk of developing fatal cancers or heritable mutations following radiation exposure. As discussed in preceding chapter, for a given absorbed dose, some organ systems such as the bone marrow and breast are more likely to develop fatal cancers than other tissues, such as cortical bone and the brain. Similarly, irradiation of gonadal organs increases the risk of transmitting a heritable mutation.

The parameter **effective dose** (E or H_e) was developed to estimate these relative risks. Although originally applied to occupational dosimetry, effective dose is increasingly being used to compare doses between different imaging modalities such as CT and nuclear medicine studies. One can think of the effective dose as a sum of all of the "tissue-weighted" organ doses for the body:

$$E = \sum_T W_T \times D_T$$

where T is a specific type of tissue, such as liver or red marrow, D_T is the absorbed dose in the tissue, and W_T is the tissue weighting factor. Table 15.4 contains standard W_T values; higher values are applied to more radiosensitive organs or tissues.

Table 15.4 Tissue weighting factors (W_T)

Tissue (T)	Number of tissues	W_T	Total contribution
Lung, stomach, colon, bone marrow, breast, remainder	6	0.12	0.72
Gonads	1	0.08	0.08
Thyroid, esophagus, bladder, liver	4	0.04	0.16
Bone surface, skin, brain, salivary glands	4	0.01	0.04
Total			**1.00**

Source: ICRP, 2007. The 2007 Recommendations of the International Commission on Radiological Protection, ICRP Publication 103, Ann. ICRP 37(2-4), p. 261.

CT dosimetry

The dose to a patient receiving a CT scan is largely dependent upon the number and energies of the X-rays produced by the X-ray tube. The greater the number of X-rays (a function of the tube current, measured in mAs) and the greater the maximum energy of the electrons (determined by the maximum voltage applied across the tube, measured in kV), the greater the patient dose. As discussed in Chapter 9, the radiation dose to the patient is somewhat reduced by filtering out the lower-energy X-rays in the spectrum. Many other scanner-based factors contribute to patient dose and include beam collimation, detector efficiency, and pitch.

Absorbed dose in CT

CTDI

Absorbed doses from CT imaging are approximated by scanning phantoms containing dosimeters. The average absorbed dose at any point in a scanned slice of a standardized phantom is approximated by the quantity **CTDI$_{vol}$** (computed tomography dose index volume), which is frequently abbreviated as "CTDI" without a suffix. CTDI is expressed in milligrays.

DLP

CTDI values estimate the dose at a point in a single slice of the phantom, but do not take the actual length of the CT scan into account. It would make sense that the patient dose from a CT scan encompassing the chest, abdomen, and pelvis would be greater than the dose from a chest CT alone or from a scan of a single slice (assuming all scans were acquired with the same technique, using the same kVp, mA s, etc.). To take the length of the

---

Derivation of CTDI$_{vol}$

The calculation of CTDI$_{vol}$ begins with measurements of doses to standard CT phantoms containing thin dosimeters. Two standard phantoms are used to measure the absorbed dose; one is larger in diameter to simulate the human torso, and a smaller phantom approximates the dimensions of the human head. One commonly used dosimeter is 100 mm long, and the total dose measurement along the length of the dosimeter after scanning a single central slice is termed **CTDI$_{100}$**. This dose comes from the X-rays that contribute to forming an image of the slice and the scattered radiation that is created in the rest of the phantom (Figure 15.3).

It was found that CTDI$_{100}$ measurements in the center of the scanned slice of the larger torso phantom were significantly less than the peripheral readings, largely as a result of attenuation of the X-rays as they traversed the acrylic medium. Therefore a modification, called **CTDI$_w$**, was devised, which is a weighted average of the peripheral and central dosimetry readings:

$$CTDI_w = (2/3) \times CTDI_{100} \text{ at periphery} + (1/3) \times CTDI_{100} \text{ at center}$$

CTDI$_{vol}$ represents a further refinement of CTDI dosimetry calculations and is obtained when CTDI$_w$ is divided by the pitch of the CT scan:

$$CTDI_{vol} = CTDI_w / pitch$$

(Continued)

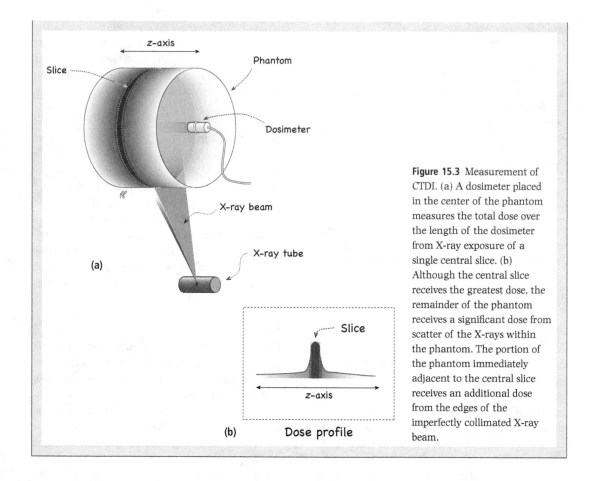

Figure 15.3 Measurement of CTDI. (a) A dosimeter placed in the center of the phantom measures the total dose over the length of the dosimeter from X-ray exposure of a single central slice. (b) Although the central slice receives the greatest dose, the remainder of the phantom receives a significant dose from scatter of the X-rays within the phantom. The portion of the phantom immediately adjacent to the central slice receives an additional dose from the edges of the imperfectly collimated X-ray beam.

study into account, another parameter, **DLP (dose length product)**, is frequently reported and is calculated as

$$DLP\,(mGy\text{-}cm) = L\,(cm) \times CTDI_{vol}\,(mGy)$$

where L is the total length of the scan.

Estimation of relative risk: effective dose

Mathematical simulations of CT scans using computerized models of a body combined with scanner-specific dose measurements are used to estimate organ doses. Then, in a similar fashion to the calculation of effective dose described in the preceding section on nuclear medicine dosimetry, these organ doses are multiplied by organ-specific weighting factors (W_T) and the results are summed to obtain the effective dose.

One simplification for estimation of the effective dose E is achieved by multiplying the DLPs for each region of the body, such as the head, chest,

abdomen, and pelvis, by region-specific conversion factors, also called **k factors** or **k conversion coefficients**. Some sample k factors are 0.0023 mSv/mGy cm for the head, 0.017 mSv/mGy cm for the chest, and 0.015 mSv/mGy cm for the abdomen [2]:

$$E\,(mSv) = DLP\,(mGy\ cm) \times k(mSv/mGy\ cm)$$

References

1. Snyder WS, Ford MR, Warner GG, Watson SB. *Absorbed Dose Per Unit Cumulated Activity for Selected Radionuclides and Organs*, MIRD Pamphlet No. 11 "S". New York: Society of Nuclear Medicine, 1975.
2. Christner JA, Kofler JM, McCollough CH. Estimating effective dose for CT using dose-length product compared with using organ doses: consequences of adopting International Commission on Radiological Protection publication 103 or dual-energy scanning. *AJR Am J Roentgenol* 2010; 194(4):881–889.

Questions

1. True or false: The effective half-life is always longer than either the physical or the biological half-life.

2. What is the effective half life of rubidium-86, which has a biological half-life of 45 days and a physical half-life of 18.8 days?

3. True or false: The biological half-life of a radiopharmaceutical labeled with ^{99m}Tc will be shorter than that of the same compound labeled with ^{111}In.

4. True or false: When calculating the total dose to a target organ, the target organ should be included as one of the radiation sources.

5. Which measurement of dosimetry can be used to compare the relative risks of fatal cancer or heritable mutations as a result of radiation exposure from different types of diagnostic studies?
   (a) Dose equivalent (H_T).
   (b) Effective dose (E).
   (c) Total absorbed dose.

6. True or false: In general, absorbed dose values for diagnostic radiologic procedures are only estimates based on computer models and phantoms.

7. Which estimate of absorbed dose for CT procedures takes the length of the CT scan into account?
   (a) CTDI.
   (b) DLP.

Answers

1. False: The effective half-life is equal to or shorter than either the physical or the biological half-life.
2. 13 days.
3. False: The biological half-life of a radiopharmaceutical is not affected by the physical half-life of the nuclide.
4. True.
5. (b).
6. True.
7. (b): DLP, or dose length product.

CHAPTER 16

Radiation Safety

Rationale

The purpose of a radiation protection program is to monitor individuals' contact with radiation and to limit their exposure to as low a level as possible. In the US, Federal regulations that outline acceptable levels of exposure are issued by the Nuclear Regulatory Commission (NRC). In addition, the government has set forth a general policy principle referred to as **ALARA**. To quote from the Federal Register, Volume 56, No. 98:

> ALARA (acronym for "as low as reasonably achievable") means making every reasonable effort to maintain exposures to radiation as far below the dose limits [...] as is practical consistent with the purpose for which the licensed activity is undertaken.

Dose limits

Radiation doses may come from radiation sources outside the body (for example, an X-ray machine or radioactive material external to the body) or from radioactive material that has been taken into the body. These two modes of exposure to radiation are called **external exposure** and **internal exposure**, respectively. Table 16.1 lists the terms commonly used to describe radiation exposure. Dose limits are prescribed separately for occupational workers (including the fetus of a pregnant worker) and the general public.

Occupational exposure

The prescribed limits for occupational exposure for radiation workers are listed in Table 16.2. Exposure limits for the embryo or fetus of a radiation worker can only be applied to workers who have voluntarily declared their pregnancy in written form.

Hospital workers

The maximal permissible exposure for hospital workers who are not classified as radiation workers is the same as for the general public: 1 mSv/year (0.1 rem/year). If an individual is likely to receive over 10% of any of the acceptable limits, they are classified as radiation workers and must be monitored (for example, by using a pen dosimeter or wearing a film and/or ring badge). For individuals receiving less than this amount, their exposure is estimated. The limit refers only to cumulative exposure from the workplace and does not include contributing doses from background radiation, any personal medical radiation exposure, etc.

Exposure for the general public

The estimated annual total effective dose equivalent (TEDE) for a member of the public should be less than 1 mSv (0.1 rem). The estimated exposure in an unrestricted area (such as a waiting room) must be less than 0.02 mSv/h (2 mrem/h). Exceptions to these limits are allowed under certain conditions for household contacts of patients receiving radioactive materials for treatment (see the section on "Limiting Exposure of Family Members and the Public"). **Background whole body radiation**, at sea level, is approximately 3.6 mSv/year (360 mrem/year), including 2.0 mSv/year (200 mrem/year) from radon.

Essentials of Nuclear Medicine Physics and Instrumentation, Third Edition. Rachel A. Powsner, Matthew R. Palmer, and Edward R. Powsner.
© 2013 John Wiley & Sons, Ltd. Published 2013 by John Wiley & Sons, Ltd.

Table 16.1 Terms used to describe radiation exposure

Term	Abbreviation	Description
Calculated		
Absorbed dose	D	Energy deposited in a unit mass of irradiated material (such as tissue) following exposure to ionizing radiation (expressed in units of Gy and rad)
Weighting factor, radiation (quality factor)	W_R (Q)	Relative biologic effectiveness of type of radiation: $W_R = 1$ for gamma, X-ray, and beta radiation, and $W_R = 20$ for alpha particles (see Chapter 14)
Dose equivalent	H_T (H)	Absorbed dose times radiation weighting factor: $H_T = D \times W_R$; for nuclear medicine exposures, $H_T = D$ (expressed in units of Sv and rem)
Weighting factor, tissue	W_T	The weighting factor for organ T is the ratio of the risk of death from stochastic effects (cancer) from irradiation of organ T to the risk of stochastic effects if the same dose was distributed uniformly over the entire body; this value reflects both the relative radiosensitivity of the organ and the risk of fatality from irradiation. For example, W_T for the thyroid is 0.04 (since thyroid cancer is generally treatable); in contrast, W_T for bone marrow is 0.12 (owing to its high radiosensitivity and the risk of leukemia). See Table 15.4 for a list of tissue weighting factors.
Effective dose (effective dose equivalent)	H_E	$H_T \times W_T$ (calculated for all exposed organs and then summed)
Committed dose equivalent	$H_{T,50}$	Dose equivalent to organ T over the 50 years following intake of a quantity of radioactivity
Committed effective dose equivalent	$H_{E,50}$	$H_{T,50} \times W_T$ (calculated for all exposed organs and then summed)
Total organ dose equivalent	TODE	Total dose to an individual organ from both internal and external exposure, equal to $H_{T,50} + H_d$ (except for the lens of the eye)
Total effective dose equivalent	TEDE	Sum of effective dose equivalent (for external exposures) and the committed effective dose equivalent (for internal exposures): TEDE $= H_E + H_{E,50}$
Measured		
Deep dose equivalent	H_d	External exposure of the whole body, as measured by a whole body radiation monitoring badge at a tissue-equivalent depth of 1 cm[a]
Shallow dose equivalent	SDE	External exposure of the skin, measured by a whole body radiation monitoring badge at a tissue-equivalent depth of 0.007 cm[a] or an extremity measured by a ring badge
Lens dose equivalent	LDE	External exposure of the lens of the eye, measured by a whole body radiation monitoring badge at a tissue-equivalent depth of 0.3 cm[a]

Source: US Nuclear Regulatory Commission. 10CFR Part 20, Standards for Protection Against Radiation, 20.1003, Definitions.

[a]Tissue depths are simulated by the use of filters placed within the case of a whole body radiation monitoring film or luminescent radiation badge; see Chapter 4 for a description of monitoring badges.

Methods for limiting exposure

Limiting occupational exposure

Limiting external exposure

The three methods of reducing external exposure relate to time, distance, and shielding.

Time: Minimize the time spent in the vicinity of a source of radiation. Work efficiently, but do not rush.

Distance: Maintain as large a distance from the source as practical. The radiation intensity from a source (patient or dose) diminishes rapidly as the distance from the source is increased. In Figure 16.1, the bird in the middle is closer to the source of the radiation (the bird on the left) and receives more radiation than the more distant bird on the right. The radiation dose decreases as the inverse square of the distance (r) from the source (i.e., as $1/r^2$). Figure 16.2 illustrates areas of equal expo-

Table 16.2 NRC radiation dose equivalent limits for occupational exposure (abridged)

Organ/system	Limit in rem/year	Limit in mSv/year
Total effective dose equivalent (TEDE)[a]	5	50
Sum of DDE and $H_{T,50}$[a] (except for lens of eye)	50	500
Lens dose equivalent (LDE)[a]	15	150
Shallow dose equivalent to skin or extremity (SDE)[a]	50	500
Dose equivalent to embryo/fetus[b]	0.5 (0.05/month)	5 (0.5/month)
Dose equivalent to minors (<18 years)[c]	10% of adult limits	10% of adult limits

[a]US Nuclear Regulatory Commission. 10CFR Part 20, Standards for Protection Against Radiation, 20.1201, Occupational dose limits for adults.
[b]US Nuclear Regulatory Commission. 10CFR Part 20, Standards for Protection Against Radiation, 20.1208, Dose equivalent to an embryo/fetus (For workers who have declared their pregnancy).
[c]US Nuclear Regulatory Commission. 10CFR Part 20, Standards for Protection Against Radiation, 20.1207, Occupational dose limits for minors.

sure at distances of r and $2r$ from a source. At a distance r, the entire dose is spread over a sphere with a surface area of $4\pi r^2$. At twice this distance ($2r$), the dose is spread over a sphere with four times the area ($16\pi r^2$); the radiation dose at twice the distance ($2r$) is equal to one-fourth of the dose at a distance r. When radioactive doses are being handled, tools such as tongs can effectively reduce exposure of hands and forearms.

Shielding: When time and distance alone are not sufficient, shielding is usually used. Shields take many forms: syringe shields, vial shields, counter-top shields (often with leaded glass), and fixed and portable (on casters) lead barriers, as well as thinner shields of plastic that may be used for beta-emitting and very low-energy gamma-emitting sources. The use of lead and other dense materials as shielding for beta particles is discouraged because the dose will be increased owing to the bremsstrahlung effect (see Chapter 2).

Limiting internal exposure

Protection techniques are oriented mainly toward preventing radioactive material from entering the body. Entrance is most commonly by inhalation, but ingestion, absorption through intact skin, and intake through skin puncture are also possible.

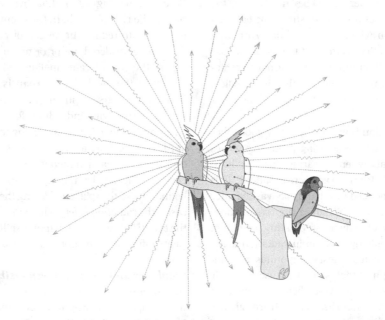

Figure 16.1 Exposure decreases as a function of distance from the source.

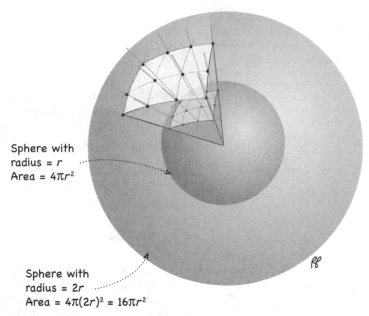

Sphere with
radius = r
Area = $4\pi r^2$

Sphere with
radius = $2r$
Area = $4\pi(2r)^2 = 16\pi r^2$

Figure 16.2 Exposure decreases as the square of the distance from the source.

Limiting inhalation is accomplished by good laboratory design, including attention to adequate air replacement and good airflow patterns; by the use of fume hoods; and by other laboratory practices developed with minimizing inhalation in mind. For example, when working with a volatile radioactive source, the worker should be "upwind" of the source, that is to say, the source should be between the worker and an exhaust such as a hood. Although obvious, this practice is often not followed. The use of respirators to limit inhalation of airborne radioactive material is almost never required in a medical institution and should be considered only as a last resort.

Limiting ingestion is accomplished by good laboratory hygiene, such as wearing protective gloves and hospital coats when preparing doses or handling body fluids from a radioactive patient. It is strongly recommended that hands be washed after the removal of gloves. To reduce the risk of inadvertent ingestion of radioactivity, eating, drinking, smoking, and applying makeup in radiation areas are strictly prohibited. Most compounds are not absorbed through intact skin. Because of their chemical composition, however, beta emitters such as ^{32}P and ^{131}I are absorbed readily through the skin. When dealing with these materials, extra

care should be taken to properly cover the hands, forearms, and other parts that could become contaminated.

Reducing the risk of contamination following a radiation spill

Careful handling of radioactive materials can reduce the risk of a spill. In the event of a spill, it is important to reduce the spread of contamination. Spills are considered minor or major spills depending on the type of radionuclide and the estimated activity of the spill [1]. **Minor spills** are controlled by notifying persons in the area that a spill has occurred, surveying individuals for contamination, cleaning up the spill, and surveying the area. **Major spills** require more aggressive measures, including clearing the area of noncontaminated individuals, covering but not cleaning up the spill, marking the boundaries of the spill, and locking the room. In both cases, the radiation safety officer must be notified of the event; in the event of a major spill, the radiation safety officer must be notified immediately [2].

Employer and employee responsibilities in controlling risk

If an employee is likely to receive more than 10% of any annual limit, the employer is required to perform monitoring. In the case of external exposure, this is usually done with a personal dosimeter such as a film badge or other type of monitor. If the exposure is likely to be internal, for example from vapors of ^{131}I, monitoring thyroidal uptake is recommended to assess contamination. If the exposure is from ^{32}P, the radiation officer must assess the body burden by measurement of urine counts. A total dose should be estimated based on the effective half-life of the radioactivity.

At least annually, employers are required to notify each monitored employee of the employee's dose. Employers also are required to notify an employee in the event that any limit has been exceeded. If an employee decides that the risks associated with occupational radiation exposure are too high, the employee may request a reassignment by the employer; however, the employer is not required to provide such a reassignment.

Employees should immediately notify their supervisor if they suspect that a work condition is unsafe or that an NRC or state regulation or a provision of the license has been violated. The NRC requires licensees to post Form NRC-3, which summarizes employee rights and responsibilities [3].

Limiting exposure of patients

Patient doses are calculated with the intention of reducing the exposure to as low a value as possible while performing a clinically useful diagnostic test or treatment. Special consideration must be given to the **pregnant patient**. The benefit of the test for the mother should be weighed against the potential risk to the fetus. In general, limited diagnostic testing is possible. The administered dose should be reduced to the lowest feasible value. **Breast-feeding** should be discontinued until there is no significant amount of radiopharmaceutical present in the breast milk, which depends on the biological distribution and effective half-life of the radiopharmaceutical. Based on a limited number of available cases, guidelines have been devised for breast-feeding mothers [4]. Breast-feeding does not need to be interrupted for some ^{99m}Tc-tagged radiopharmaceuticals such as ^{99m}Tc-MDP, but a 13 h interruption is recommended for ^{99m}Tc-MAA and a 24 h interruption for ^{99m}Tc-pertechnetate. Complete cessation is recommended following administration of ^{131}I-iodide [4].

Limiting exposure of family members and the public

Education of patients and their family members is important, particularly following the administration of beta emitters such as ^{131}I and ^{89}Sr. ^{131}I and ^{89}Sr are excreted through bodily fluids, predominantly via urine. To limit exposure to family members and members of the general public, patients must be carefully instructed on how to reduce contamination. Hygienic precautions, such as flushing the toilet twice after use, hand washing, and separate laundering of clothes and linen are necessary to prevent contact with radioactive urine, sweat, and saliva. In addition, following administration of ^{131}I, which emits high-energy gammas, patients and family must be educated on the rules of time and distance, as outlined above. Patients and family members should be given written guidelines on the preceding precautions for reference after treatment.

Household contacts of patients receiving radioactive material should not receive more than 5 mSv (500 mrem) total effective dose equivalent from exposure to the patient. For children or pregnant women, this limit is 1 mSv (100 mrem) [5]. Previously, to ensure exposures did not exceed these values, hospital admission was required for doses of ^{131}I sodium iodide that equaled or exceeded 1110 MBq (30 mCi). Patients can now receive higher activities as outpatients if, using dose calculations, it can be shown that the total effective dose equivalent for household contacts will not exceed 5 mSv (1 mSv for children and pregnant women). The procedure for calculating doses is outlined in NUREG-1556, Vol. 9 Rev. 2 [6].

In general, though, hospitalization is still recommended for incontinent patients or patients who cannot care for themselves. The hospital rooms used for admission must be designated for radiation therapy and be monitored by the radiation safety staff to reduce staff, visitor, and other patient exposure.

Regulations

The NRC regulations pertaining to the above text and other standard procedures performed in the routine practice of nuclear medicine are summarized in Appendix D.

References

1. US Nuclear Regulatory Commission. NUREG-1556, Vol. 9, Appendix N, Table N.1, Relative hazards of common radionuclides. In: *Consolidated Guidance about Materials Licenses: Program-Specific Guidance about Medical Use Licenses*, January 2008.

2. US Nuclear Regulatory Commission. NUREG-1556, Vol. 9, Appendix N, Model emergency procedures. In: *Consolidated Guidance about Materials Licenses: Program-Specific Guidance about Medical Use Licenses*, January 2008.

3. Powsner ER, Widman JC. Basic principles of radioactivity and its measurement. In: Burtis C, Ashwood E (eds.) *Tietz Textbook of Clinical Chemistry*, 3rd edn. Philadelphia: WB Saunders, 1998.

4. US Nuclear Regulatory Commission. US NRC Regulatory Guide 8.39, *Release of Patients Administered Radioactive Materials*, April 1997.

5. US Nuclear Regulatory Commission. NRC Regulation 10, Part 35.75, *Release of Individuals Containing Unsealed byproduct Material or Implants Containing Byproduct Material*, November 2012.

6. US Nuclear Regulatory Commission. NUREG-1556, Vol. 9, Appendix U, Model procedure for release of patients or human research subjects administered radioactive materials. In: *Consolidated Guidance about Materials Licenses: Program-Specific Guidance about Medical Use Licenses*, January 2008.

Questions

1. Associate the following annual exposures with the permissible maximum doses:
   (a) TEDE, total effective dose equivalent, for a member of the public.
   (b) Maximum permissible exposure for a hospital worker who is not a radiation worker.
   (c) Background whole body radiation at sea level.
   (d) Maximum permissible TEDE for a radiation worker.
      (i) 50 mSv (5.0 rem).
      (ii) 3.6 mSv (0.36 rem).
      (iii) 1.0 mSv (0.1 rem).

2. Select the three most effective ways to reduce exposure when working with radioactivity.
   (a) Reduce the time spent in the vicinity of a radioactive source.
   (b) Use soap when washing your hands.
   (c) Maintain the maximum possible distance from the source.
   (d) Shield the radioactive source.
   (e) Wear a face mask.

3. A nursing mother should be instructed to permanently discontinue breast-feeding under which of the following circumstances?
   (a) After receiving any radiopharmaceutical.
   (b) After receiving an injection of ^{67}Ga citrate.
   (c) After receiving an injection of 37 MBq of ^{99m}Tc-MAA.
   (d) After ingesting 370 MBq of ^{131}I.

4. True or false: The maximum allowable exposure for the household contacts of a patient receiving radioactivity, including children and pregnant women, is 5 mSv.

5. True or false: Radionuclide spills are classified as either major or minor spills based on the volume of fluid involved.

6. The embryo/fetus dose equivalent limits for radiation workers can be applied under which conditions?
   (a) For a radiation worker who is obviously pregnant but who has not declared her pregnancy in written form.
   (b) For a radiation worker who has declared her pregnancy in written form.
   (c) Both (a) and (b).

7. Bob is standing 1 m away from a radioactive source; Phyllis is standing 2 m away from the same source. Neither is shielded. Which of the following is true about Phyllis's exposure compared with Bob's exposure?
   (a) Phyllis's radiation exposure is equal to Bob's.
   (b) Phyllis's radiation exposure is half of Bob's.
   (c) Phyllis's radiation exposure is one-quarter of Bob's.

8. If the exposure rate for a point source is 1 R/h at 1 m, what is the exposure rate at 3 m?
   (a) 3 R/h.
   (b) 0.33 R/h.
   (c) 0.25 R/h.
   (d) 0.11 R/h.

Answers

1. (a) (iii). (b) (iii). (c) (ii). (d) (i).
2. (a), (c), (d).
3. (d).
4. False: It is 5 mSv for everyone except for children and pregnant women, for whom the limit is 1 mSv.
5. False: The activity and type of radionuclide determine whether a spill is major or minor.
6. (b).
7. (c).
8. (d). Exposure varies with the square of the distance from the source, so three times the distance means a reduction by a factor of 9.

CHAPTER 17

Management of Nuclear Event Casualties

Rachel A. Powsner, Edward R. Powsner and *Kevin Donohoe*[1]

[1]Beth Israel Deaconess Medical Center and Harvard Medical School, Boston, USA

Recent events have raised awareness of the need for hospital personnel to be prepared to evaluate and treat irradiated and/or contaminated victims of unexpected hazardous nuclear events. In any unexpected exposure to ionizing radiation, the person exposed may or may not be aware of the exposure. If the amount of exposure is small, the person is unlikely to experience any adverse health effects, and if the person is unaware of the exposure, they will not report to a hospital for treatment. In the unlikely event that an unknown exposure is substantial, the exposed individual may develop generalized symptoms that may be mistaken for another illness. These patients pose a diagnostic dilemma for the health care team and unless the possibility of radiation exposure is considered, the diagnosis will be delayed, if made at all. In the case of a publicized exposure event, it is likely that the number of people seeking assistance who were not exposed (but concerned that they might have been) will be much greater than the number who actually were exposed. Because the number of people who were not exposed can easily overwhelm any health care system designed to treat acutely ill patients, it is important to plan not only for treatment of the injured but also for triage of the "worried well."

This chapter begins with a brief discussion of the interaction of radiation with tissue. This is followed by a section on facility preparation for decontamination and treatment of victims of a radiation accident. A discussion of clinical techniques for early dose assessment for appropriate triage is followed by a review of the acute radiation syndromes. The chapter concludes with an introduction to the treatment of internal contamination.

Interaction of radiation with tissue

Although exposure to neutrons is virtually never encountered in the practice of clinical nuclear medicine, it must be considered a possibility during accidents or terrorist events. With this in mind, the discussion of the interaction of radiation with tissue has been expanded to include neutron radiation.

Alpha particles

Alpha particles have a charge of +2 and a weight of 4 amu. Because they are relatively heavy and charged, they have a short range in matter and a high LET (see Chapter 3). They travel only a few centimeters in air and only about $50\,\mu m$ in tissue. A few layers of dead skin readily block alpha particles, and they therefore can not damage intact skin (Figure 17.1). On the other hand, the linings of the gastrointestinal and pulmonary systems are not covered by dead cells and are susceptible to damage from direct contact with ingested or inhaled alpha-emitting atoms (Figure 17.2). The high LET of alpha particles means that all of their radiation energy is deposited within these lining cells. Furthermore, rapid cell turnover in tissues such as bronchial or gastrointestinal epithelium means that a greater proportion of cells are in a state of mitosis, which makes them relatively more vulnerable to radiation injury (see Chapter 14).

Essentials of Nuclear Medicine Physics and Instrumentation, Third Edition. Rachel A. Powsner, Matthew R. Palmer, and Edward R. Powsner.

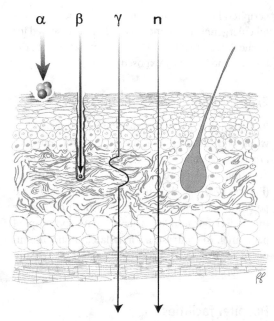

Figure 17.1 Alpha particles are stopped by layers of dead epidermis; high-energy beta particles can penetrate short distances into skin; gamma photons and neutrons can penetrate into deep tissue.

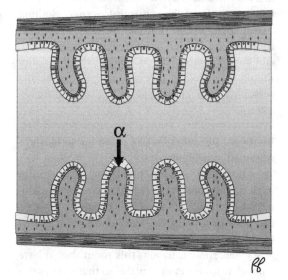

Figure 17.2 Alpha particles can damage the lining epithelium of the gastrointestinal tract or pulmonary system.

Beta particles

Beta particles have a charge of −1 and a mass of 0.00055 amu. They have a lower LET and therefore penetrate matter farther than alpha particles of the same energy; they can travel as far as a few meters

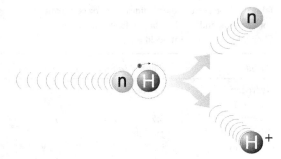

Figure 17.3 Elastic scattering of a proton following interaction of a neutron with a hydrogen atom nucleus.

in air and a few millimeters in tissue. Because they can penetrate the dead skin layer of the epithelium, beta particles may be responsible for radiation-induced skin burns. Beta emitters, like all radiation, can also do significant cell injury if ingested or inhaled in sufficient amounts.

Gamma rays and X-rays

Photons have no charge and no mass, and therefore they have relatively few interactions with surrounding matter or air. Gamma and X-ray photons can travel several kilometers in air and penetrate deeply into or through tissues. If these photons interact with tissues, they may cause both superficial and deep tissue injury.

Neutrons

Neutrons are different from the preceding types of radiation in a number of ways. They have a finite existence, with a half-life of 12 min in air, following which they decay into a proton, electron, and neutrino. They have a mass of 1 amu and no charge. Since they have no positive or negative charge, they lack the great attractive or repulsive forces in their interactions with atoms that we have seen with charged particles (alphas and betas). For this reason, as well as differences in mass, the interactions of neutrons with atoms are limited to atomic nuclei. Also, like photons, neutrons can penetrate and pass through tissue; they differ from photons in that they have mass and, as a result, can interact directly with the hydrogen nuclei in tissue through a process called **elastic scattering** (Figure 17.3). In this process, some of the kinetic energy of the neutron is transferred to the proton and the proton is separated from its atom. The proton thus becomes

Table 17.1 Selected radionuclides used for occupational applications and/or identified in fallout from the Chernobyl power plant accident

Nuclide	Physical half-life	Emissions
Hydrogen-3 (tritium)	12 years	β^-
Carbon-14	5.7×10^3 years	β^-
Phosphorus-32	14.3 days	β^-
Cobalt-60	5.27 years	β^-, γ
Strontium-90	28 years	β^-
Iodine-125	60.1 days	γ
Iodine-131	8 days	β^-, γ
Cesium-137	30 years	β^-, γ
Iridium-192	74 days	β^-
Uranium-235	7×10^8 years	α, γ
Uranium-238	4.5×10^9 years	α, γ
Plutonium-238	88 years	α, γ
Plutonium-239	2.4×10^4 years	α, γ
Americium-241	458 years	α

Derived in part from Soloviev et al. [1], UNSCEAR [2], and REAC/TS [3].

a moving charged particle, which can damage surrounding tissue. Exposure to neutrons can result in both superficial and deep tissue injury.

Radionuclides

The radionuclides that are more commonly used for research, military, or industrial applications, as well as some of the nuclides that were identified in radioactive fallout from the Chernobyl nuclear power plant accident, are listed in Table 17.1.

Hospital response to a radiation accident

In the event of a large radiation accident, there may be large numbers of people presenting to hospitals for evaluation, and past experience tells us it is likely that the majority of these individuals will be uninjured. Screening a large number of otherwise well individuals for contamination and possible radiation exposure can overwhelm limited hospital resources, which are needed to treat injured patients. Establishing a **screening and decontamination facility** at an off-site location and redirecting people to that location may be a solution to this problem. Alternatively, an on-site decontamination facility separate from the hospital, such as a large tent or a

peripheral building, may suffice. A prepared hospital emergency department can then be reserved for medical treatment and decontamination of the injured and critically exposed.

Exposure and contamination

Radiation accidents can result in partial body or whole body irradiation. If aerosolized radionuclides are released during the accident, an individual's skin and/or clothing can become **contaminated** (Figure 17.4(a)). A contaminated individual is a potential source of radiation exposure not only for themselves but also for other patients and hospital personnel. In contrast, an irradiated, noncontaminated person is NOT a source of radiation exposure for others (Figure 17.4(b)).

Hospital facilities

Decontamination facility

In preparation for a large number of contaminated but well individuals, some hospitals have designated an area such as a tent or a peripheral hospital building with easily controlled access, clothing collection hampers, multiple showers with large wastewater collection tanks, replacement clothing, and survey meters. When needed, these facilities should be staffed by properly clothed (see below) personnel with knowledge of the use of survey meters.

Treatment/Decontamination room for seriously wounded individuals

The treatment of life-threatening wounds or medical conditions takes priority over decontamination. Patients with these conditions may be cared for in a previously designated combination treatment/decontamination room in the emergency department. Ideally, this room should have immediate access to the outside so that transportation of a contaminated individual into the room does not risk contamination of the rest of the emergency department. A **buffer zone** should be established for decontamination and monitoring of personnel and patients leaving the treatment room prior to entering the rest of the hospital. If there is adequate notification prior to patient arrival, the treatment room may be prepared with a secure floor covering with a nonskid surface to aid in room

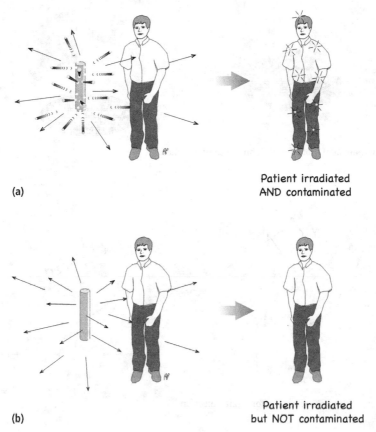

(a)

Patient irradiated
AND contaminated

(b)

Patient irradiated
but NOT contaminated

Figure 17.4 Exposure and contamination.

decontamination. Several large plastic-lined waste containers should be present, and any equipment present in the room that is not needed should be covered to help prevent contamination. A shielded area or a location away from the treatment area should be identified for containment of solid radioactive debris such as shrapnel from a wound. A pair of long-handled tongs for handling metal fragments should be available. After the patient is medically stabilized, decontamination can proceed.

External decontamination

Although the standard practice of having emergency room or ambulance personnel remove a victim's clothing will often accomplish the majority of the surface decontamination, further cleaning may be required. Prior to decontamination, swab samples of contaminated areas should be obtained

and placed in carefully labeled plastic specimen tubes for later analysis.

Decontamination should proceed in the following order: wounds, orifices, and intact skin. Contaminated wounds can be flushed with water; however, using a damp washcloth or even the application of minimal water will help to avoid spreading contamination and producing large volumes of contaminated fluids. Draping the area around the wound will prevent contamination of surrounding skin. Abrasion of skin or wounds is contraindicated, to minimize absorption of superficial contamination.

If contaminated, the eyes and ears can be gently flushed with water or saline; oral cavity contamination can be reduced by repeated rinsing and by brushing teeth. The nasal cavity can usually be cleared by simply having the patient blow his/her nose. Shampooing hair with gentle shampoos

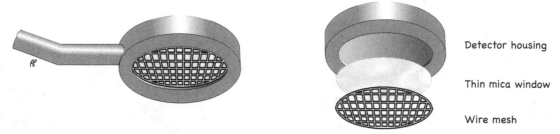

Figure 17.5 Frisking (pancake) probe for attachment to survey meter.

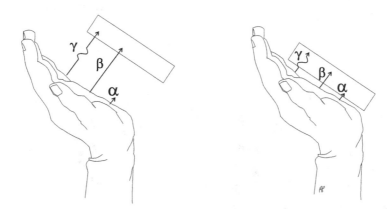

Figure 17.6 Detector proximity is necessary for alpha detection.

without conditioners prior to skin washing is recommended. Conditioners are problematic, as they bind particles to hair.

The use of soft cloths and lukewarm water and soap is recommended for skin cleansing; alternatively, diaper wipes or equivalent can be used. Cleansing of the skin should be gentle; abrading the skin may increase absorption of contaminants, and damage to irradiated skin may delay healing.

Patient radiation survey

Following removal of clothing and prior to decontamination, the patient should be **surveyed** to provide a baseline measurement of contamination. When performing surveys, it is important to move the probe slowly and to keep a fixed distance from the body. If possible, careful records of the distribution of contamination and of readings at sites of contamination should be made.

Following washing, the survey should be repeated using the same distance as used for the earlier survey. Decontamination should proceed until no

more contamination can be removed, and should be stopped if the skin becomes irritated. Skin that remains contaminated can be swathed in plastic to encourage sweating to remove additional local contamination. The plastic should be removed periodically and the area redressed as needed.

Survey meter

A standard **Geiger–Müller survey meter** (see Chapter 4) with a **frisking** or **pancake probe** (Figure 17.5) is adequate for monitoring the progress of decontamination. The very thin mica window behind the protective wire mesh allows detection of gamma photons, alpha particles, and some beta particles.

This method of surveying is limited by the inability of **low-energy betas** (with energies lower than 60 keV), such as those from tritium, to penetrate the mica [4]. Although most commonly encountered **alpha particles** are of high enough kinetic energy to penetrate the mica window (>3 MeV), alpha particles have a short range in air and can only be detected with the probe placed very close to the area to be surveyed (Figure 17.6). However, one must not actually touch the surface, to avoid contamination of the probe itself. Covering the probe with a glove to prevent its contamination may also block alpha particles and prevent their detection. Probes are available that are more efficient for the detection of alpha particles and low-energy beta particles, but most hospitals do not have such specialized detectors available.

Survey meter quality control

Prior to use, a battery check and source check should be performed on the survey meter. The inspection sticker on the side of the meter should be checked to verify that the yearly calibration is up to date. For more detailed information on the calibration of survey meters, see Chapter 13.

A rough **discrimination of alpha, beta, and gamma emissions** can be performed by comparing the reading directly from the source with that obtained with an intervening piece of paper to block alpha particles and then with an intervening piece of aluminum or plastic to block both alpha and beta particles (Figure 17.7).

Personnel

Personal protection

Wearing protective coverings will greatly reduce the risk of contamination of hospital staff involved in patient care. Caps or hoods (particularly for individuals with long hair), eye protection, masks, gowns, double gloves (with the inner glove taped to the gown sleeve), and plastic shoe covers are recommended for personnel directly involved with decontamination. Plastic is preferable to paper for shoe covers for its durability and resistance to liquids. Gowning and gloving with materials that are readily available in the surgical suite is often perfectly acceptable. Using standard surgical clothing also ensures that the clothing needed is always available and in adequate supply.

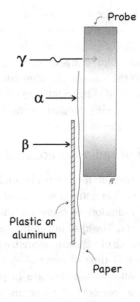

Figure 17.7 Paper and plastic or aluminum can be placed between the radioactive source and the detector to aid in differentiating alpha, beta, and gamma emissions.

If there is a credible risk of contamination from radioactive iodine (^{131}I), medical personnel should be treated with oral potassium iodide as soon as possible prior to exposure to radioiodine.

Reducing exposure

The standard practices for minimizing total exposure are reducing the **time** of exposure, increasing the **distance** from the source of the radiation, and, when feasible, placing **shielding** between the radiation source and personnel. These fundamentals remain applicable when treating radiation accident victims. When heavily contaminated patients are being treated, staff should be rotated to reduce the time any one individual spends with the patient, if possible. When not directly caring for a contaminated patient, staff should try to remain a reasonable distance away from the patient. Historically, hospital-based medical personnel treating radiation accident victims, including those who treated victims from the Chernobyl accident, received only minimal radiation exposures.

Dosimeters

Personnel should be supplied with direct reading dosimeters, such as pocket dosimeters, so that immediate readings are available at the time of exposure. Depending on the device used, however, these devices may not provide a means of permanent record keeping and may not discriminate between types or energies of radiation. All personnel should therefore wear film badges, thermoluminescent dosimeters (TLDs), or optically stimulated luminescent detectors (OSLs) in addition to direct reading dosimeters. For a more detailed description of these devices, please refer to Chapter 4.

Evaluation of radiation accident victim

An initial history of the event obtained from the victim or a credible witness is essential for understanding the radiation exposure and the extent of medical trauma. The distance from the radiation source at the time of exposure, evidence of trauma, and the type and time of onset of symptoms are examples of information that are helpful during initial triage of patients. If radiation exposure is suspected, a complete blood count with differential, blood for **HLA typing**, urinalysis, and skin, oral, nasal, and wound swabs, as well as urine and fecal samples, should be obtained as soon as possible. The **initial lymphocyte counts** can be used with subsequent counts, obtained every 6 h, to estimate the absorbed dose. HLA typing can be used for future transfusions and stem cell or bone marrow transplants, if needed. The swabs and the blood, urine, and fecal samples can be used to estimate the quantity and type of internal contamination. A 24 h postexposure blood sample should be sent for analysis of **lymphocyte chromosomal abnormalities** for more accurate dosimetry.

The symptoms and medical course of an accident victim are determined by the type of radiation, the absorbed radiation dose, the distribution of the absorbed dose (whole body versus localized), and the route of exposure (external or internal). For example, exposure of intact skin, which is protected by several layers of dead skin cells, to a nonabsorbable alpha emitter causes relatively little injury, whereas ingestion of the same quantity of material can be fatal. Similarly, a single exposure of 10 Gy of gamma radiation to the hand will result in severe local burns and tissue damage but survival is likely; a whole body dose of 10 Gy from a gamma emitter will be lethal.

Early estimation of whole body radiation exposure
It is important to identify those patients requiring hospital admission, monitoring, and treatment following radiation exposure. Radiation survey measurements from the site of the radiation accident, patient symptoms and time of onset, and blood lymphocyte counts can be used to estimate absorbed doses.

Symptoms and time of onset following exposure
An absorbed whole body dose greater than approximately 1 Gy may cause **radiation sickness** characterized by specific signs and symptoms. The severity of the signs and symptoms and the rapidity of their onset increase with increasing absorbed dose. The most commonly sought data for early estimation of absorbed dose is the time of onset of **nausea and vomiting** following the radiation accident. Unfortunately, nausea and vomiting are also commonly seen in people involved in a sudden traumatic event who have not been exposed to radiation. These symptoms may be caused by abdominal or head trauma or merely by anxiety surrounding the event. It is important that the treating physician be made aware that exposure to radiation occurred so that they can consider the importance of the symptoms. Table 17.2 summarizes the signs and symptoms of radiation sickness and the recommended patient disposition for increasing estimated whole body doses.

Blood count estimates of exposure
Neutrophil, platelet, and lymphocyte counts decrease following radiation exposure. Lymphocytes are relatively more radiosensitive, and their counts drop more rapidly following exposure. There are several techniques for estimating dose from lymphocyte counts obtained in the early hours or days following exposure. Dose can be estimated from the minimal lymphocyte count within the first 48 h following exposure [7], from a plot of the lymphocyte counts from frequent sampling during the first 12 h after exposure [8], or from the percentage drop in the lymphocyte counts in the first 24 h [3]. It should be noted, for all dose estimates based on white blood cell counts and particularly those based on a single measurement, that lymphocyte and neutrophil counts can be adversely affected by many factors, including stress and underlying illness.

Table 17.2 Signs, symptoms, and recommended disposition of exposed patients

Estimated whole body dose (Gy)	Onset of vomiting	Percentage of cases	Diarrhea severity and onset	Percentage of cases
<1	None	–	None	–
1–2	>2 h	10–50	None	–
2–4	1–2 h	70–90	None	–
4–6	<1 h	100	Mild 3–8 h	<10
6–8	<30 min	100	Heavy 1–3 h	>10
>8	<10 min	100	Heavy <1 h	100

Estimated whole body dose (Gy)	Headache severity and time of onset	Percentage of cases	Fever	Percentage of cases	Level of consciousness
<1	None	–	None	–	Normal
1–2	Slight	–	None	–	Normal
2–4	Mild	–	Mild 1–3 h	10–80	Normal
4–6	Moderate 4–24 h	50	Moderate to high 1–2 h	80–100	Normal
6–8	Severe 3–4 h	80	High <1 h	100	May be reduced
>8	Severe 1–2 h	80–90	High <1 h	100	Unconscious—may be for only seconds or minutes (at greater than 50 Gy, incidence is 100%)

Estimated whole body dose (Gy)	Recommended disposition
<1	Outpatient with 5 week follow-up of blood labs, skin examinations
1–2	Outpatient with antiemetic therapy, and frequent laboratory and physical examination follow-up or general admission for symptomatic treatment and observation
2–4	Admission with supportive care and hematology consult[a]
4–6	Admission to tertiary care facility with intensive supportive care, including fluid management, hematology care, and infectious disease consults
6–8	Same
>8	Likely lethal, although with intense medical support may survive up to 12 Gy exposure

Adapted with permission from IAEA [5], with additional information from Cosset *et al.* [6].

[a]For estimated whole body doses greater than 3 Gy, early treatment with colony-stimulating factors is recommended [3].

Chromosomal aberrations

Quantitation of chromosomal aberrations in lymphocytes is considered to be the most reliable biologic marker for dosimetry measurements. These tests, although highly accurate for estimating exposures, are not widely available and can take several days to complete. However, techniques for more rapid assessment of chromosomal aberrations with adequate dose estimate accuracy have been developed [3].

Triage dose estimate

In order to estimate whether an externally irradiated patient has received more than 1 Gy whole body dose and should be referred for further evaluation, a simple formula has been developed by REAC/TS based on the percentage neutrophil and lymphocyte counts and the presence or absence of vomiting [3]. Using a blood sample obtained between 4 h and 2 weeks postexposure, the following equation was proposed:

$$T = N/L + E$$

where T is the triage score, N is the percentage of neutrophils, L is the percentage of lymphocytes, and E (emesis) is 0 if the patient has not vomited and 2 if the patient has vomited. A T value greater than or equal to 3.7 means that the patient should be referred for further evaluation.

Early estimation of local radiation exposure

The early biologic consequences of radiation exposure of a portion of the body or the whole body can be helpful in determining the radiation dose. The time of onset of **initial erythema** of the skin (so called to distinguish it from the later episodes of more intense reddening of the skin) can be used to estimate the absorbed local dose and guide subsequent patient management. Table 17.3 summarizes the findings.

Acute radiation sickness

Acute radiation sickness following whole body exposure is often divided into four stages. The **prodromal stage** (or prodromal syndrome) includes symptoms of anorexia, nausea, vomiting, and easy fatiguability. The greater the dose, the shorter the duration of the prodromal stage, but the more severe the symptoms. Immediate diarrhea, fever, headache, and hypertension are seen only for doses above the lethal threshold. During the **latent period**, the patient may have few or no symptoms in the presence of ongoing organ damage. **Manifest illness** is marked by symptoms related to the organ involved (see the syndromes listed below). The **recovery phase** may extend from weeks to

Table 17.3 Estimated local radiation dose and recommended patient management based on time of onset of early erythema

Estimated skin dose (Gy)	Time of onset of initial erythema and/or abnormal skin sensation	Recommended patient management
<6	None[a]	Outpatient with 5 week follow-up of blood labs and examinations
6–8	1–2 days[a]	
8–15	12–24 h	Admission to general ward for observation
15–30	8–15 h	Admission to surgical burn ward with hematology consult
>30	3–6 h. Edema of mucosa can also be seen	Admission to tertiary care facility with intensive surgical (burn) and hematology support

Adapted with permission from IAEA [5].
[a]Mettler and Upton [9], p. 288.

years if the radiation dose is not acutely lethal. The overall duration of these stages is dependent on the dose the patient received and the specific tissue that has been injured.

Acute radiation syndromes

The course of illness following exposure to a single whole body dose of greater than 2 Gy is directly related to the absorbed dose. The acute radiation syndromes may be divided into three categories:
1. Hematopoietic: doses greater than 1–2 Gy.
2. Gastrointestinal: doses greater than 6–8 Gy.
3. Central nervous system (CNS) and cardiovascular: doses greater than 20 Gy.

Hematopoietic syndrome
The prodrome consists of nausea, vomiting, diarrhea, headache, fever, and possible decreased level of consciousness presenting within 6 h of exposure and lasting days. During the latent period of 2–3 weeks, the patient will feel relatively well, but the number of circulating red blood cells, white blood cells, and platelets will be steadily decreasing. Following the latent phase, the manifest illness is characterized by infection and hemorrhage.

Gastrointestinal syndrome
The prodrome consists of the same symptoms of acute radiation sickness as seen in the hematopoietic syndrome, with a nearly universal decrease in level of consciousness beginning within minutes of exposure and lasting days. Latency is approximately one week long, during which time the patient feels relatively well. However, during the latency period the intestinal tract lining is sloughing, which leads to the manifest gastrointestinal illness stage, when the patient is likely to expire from fluid loss, electrolyte imbalance, and sepsis.

Central nervous system and cardiovascular syndrome
The patient will suffer nearly immediate nausea, vomiting, hypotension, ataxia, convulsions, and loss of consciousness. There is no latency period, and death is likely within days.

Treatment of acute radiation sickness
Approximately 50% of those patients who are exposed to an acute whole body dose of 3.5 Gy will succumb within 2 months without medical treatment ($LD_{50/60}$); with intensive medical treat-

ment, 50% survival may be achieved after exposure to as much as 8 Gy [3]. For doses above 2 Gy, hospitalization with isolation and close observation is recommended. The medical management of acute radiation sickness requires a multidisciplinary approach. Specialists in burn care, intensive care, infectious diseases, hematology, and radiation safety often need to be closely involved in patient care.

Treatment of internal contamination

Patients can become contaminated internally with radiation by ingestion, inhalation, or absorption of specific nuclides through intact skin or open wounds. Internal contamination with radiation is treated by blocking gastrointestinal absorption, blocking organ-specific uptake of the radionuclide, and/or promoting excretion of the contaminants. The treatment is directed at the element and is independent of the specific isotope of that element. For example, the treatment for ingestion of all isotopes of strontium is the same. The process of reducing the amount of internal contamination is sometimes referred to as **decorporation**. Examples of decorporation include the use of chelating agents such CaDTPA for binding plutonium (the chelated compound is more readily excreted in urine), increasing oral intake of water to dilute and increase urinary excretion of tritium, and the ingestion of potassium iodide soon after exposure to radioactive iodine to block thyroid uptake of the radionuclide. A detailed table of treatment procedures for internal contamination can be found in [10].

Local radiation injury to the skin

The clinical signs of local radiation injury to the skin may be similar to those of thermal burns, but the time of onset is dose-dependent. The time of onset of the initial erythema, which may be accompanied by pruritus, can be within 24 h following a single dose of more than 8 Gy and is usually nonexistent following a dose of less than 6 Gy (see Table 17.3). This initial erythema persists for approximately one week and is likely due to release of vasoactive amines. The manifest illness stage, i.e., intense reddening and pruritus, presents at 2–3 weeks (sooner at higher doses) following exposure and is likely due to blood vessel damage. This phase persists for 20–30 days [9].

Two characteristic skin findings following radiation exposure at higher doses are dry desquamation and wet desquamation. **Dry desquamation** is a reddened, dry, flaking, itchy skin due to partial damage to the basal layer. It occurs at a dose of 8–12 Gy, typically 25–30 days following exposure. **Moist desquamation** is characterized by blistering, redness, pain, and a weeping discharge resulting from complete damage to the basal layer of the skin. Moist desquamation begins on day 20–28 at a dose range of 15–20 Gy [5].

References

1. Soloviev V, Ilyin L, Baranov A, Guskova A, Nadejina NM. Radiation accidents in the former U.S.S.R. In: Gusev IA, Guskova AK, Mettler FA (eds.) *Medical Management of Radiation Accidents*, 2nd edn. Boca Raton, FL: CRC Press, 2001, pp. 157–165.
2. United Nations Scientific Committee on the Effects of Atomic Radiation (UNSCEAR). 2000 Report to the General Assembly, Vol. II: *Effects*, Table 2, p. 519.
3. Oak Ridge Institute for Science and Education. *The Medical Aspects of Radiation Incidents*. Oak Ridge, TN: Radiation Emergency Assistance Center/Training Site (REAC/TS), http://www.orise.orau.gov/reacts, revised 4/19/2011.
4. Steinmeyer PR. G-M Pancake detectors: everything you've wanted to know (but were afraid to ask). *RSO Mag* 2005; 10(5):7.
5. International Atomic Energy Agency. *Diagnosis and Treatment of Radiation Injuries*. Safety Report Series, No. 2. Vienna: IAEA, 1998, http://www-pub.iaea.org/MTCD/publications/PDF/P040_scr.pdf.
6. Cosset JM, Girinsky T, Helfre S, Gourmelon P. Medical management during the prodromal and latent periods. In: Ricks RC, Berger ME, O'Hara FM (eds.) *The Medical Basis for Radiation-Accident Preparedness: The Clinical Care of Victims*, Proceedings of the Fourth International REAC/TS Conference on the Medical Basis for Radiation-Accident Preparedness, March 2001. New York: Parthenon, 2002, pp. 45–51.
7. Mettler FA, Voelz GL. Major radiation exposure—What to expect and how to respond. *New England J Med* 2002; 346(20):1554–1561.
8. Goans RE, Holloway EC, Berger ME, Ricks RC. Early dose assessment in criticality accidents. *Health Phys* 2001; 81(4):446–449.
9. Mettler FA, Upton AC. *Medical Effects of Ionizing Radiation*, 3rd edn. Philadelphia: W.B. Saunders, 2008, Chapter 6.
10. International Atomic Energy Agency. *Generic Procedures for Medical Response during a Nuclear or Radiological Emergency*. Vienna: IAEA, 2005, pp. 70–72.

Questions

1. True or false: Removing clothing and washing with soap and water generally removes the majority of external radioactive contamination.

2. Which of the following are true about the interaction of neutrons with matter?
   (a) They have a positive charge, so they interact with outer-shell electrons.
   (b) Like photons, they can pass through matter without transferring energy.
   (c) The neutron can transfer some of its kinetic energy to a proton, causing its ejection from the atom.

3. True or false: A patient who has been irradiated by photons, but not contaminated, is still a radiation risk for hospital staff.

4. When using a Geiger counter with a pancake probe as a survey meter for unknown contaminants, which of the following practices are recommended?
   (a) A battery check should be performed prior to use.
   (b) Keep the probe at least one meter away from the patient or object being surveyed.
   (c) Ascertain that the meter calibration is up to date.
   (d) Place a glove over the pancake probe to prevent contamination of the probe.

5. Which of the following is true about the use of a Geiger survey meter fitted with a thin mica window?
   (a) It can be used to detect most of the commonly encountered alpha particles.
   (b) Only lower-energy beta particles (less than 60 keV) can be detected.

6. What are effective ways to reduce your total exposure when working with a radioactive patient?
   (a) When not actually tending the patient, try to keep as close to the patient as possible.
   (b) When feasible, keep radiation shielding between yourself and the patient.
   (c) Try to reduce the total amount of time you spend near the patient.
   (d) All of the above.

7. Which of the following clinical findings have been used for an initial radiation dose estimate for an accident victim?
   (a) The time of onset of nausea and vomiting.
   (b) Chest pain.
   (c) Lymphocyte counts within the first 48 h.
   (d) Time of onset of initial skin erythema.
   (e) Palpitations.
   (f) Presence of fever.

8. Associate the following statements with the appropriate acute radiation syndrome:
   (a) Occurs at absorbed doses greater than 20 Gy.
   (b) A 2–3 week latency period during which the patient's blood counts are decreasing.
   (c) No discernible latency period, and death usually occurs within days of exposure.
   (d) A one-week latency followed by fluid loss, electrolyte imbalance, and sepsis.

   Syndrome:
   (1) Hematopoietic syndrome.
   (2) Gastrointestinal syndrome.
   (3) CNS and cardiovascular syndrome.
   (4) Pulmonary–hepatic syndrome.

Answers

1. True.
2. (b) and (c).
3. False.
4. (a) and (c) are correct. The probe should be used close to but not touching the skin or object, to allow detection of alpha and beta particles. A glove will block detection of alpha particles, so it should not be used to cover the probe.

5. (a) only. (b) is not correct, as only beta particles with energies higher than 60 keV can be detected.
6. (b) and (c). (a) is incorrect; when not tending the patient, increase the distance between yourself and the patient.
7. (a), (c), (d), and (f).
8. (a) (3). (b) (1). (c) (3). (d) (2).

APPENDIX A

Common Nuclides

Nuclide	Production method	Half-life	Decay mode	$E_{\beta\,avg}$ (keV)	γ photon energies (keV)	Decay abundance	Decay product	Half-life of product
^{99m}Tc	^{99}Mo → ^{99m}Tc	6 h	IT, γ	–	**140**	0.88	^{99}Tc	2.1×10^5 years
^{67}Ga	^{66}Zn(d,n)^{67}Ga	78 h	EC, γ	–	**93**	0.38	^{67}Zn	Stable
					185	0.20		
					300	0.17		
					393	0.05		
^{111}In	^{109}Ag(α,2n)^{111}In	67 h	EC, γ	–	23	0.70	^{111}Cd	Stable
					172	0.90		
					245	0.94		
^{131}I	^{235}U(n,f)^{131}I	8 days	β⁻, γ	**284.1**	80	0.06	^{131}Xe	Stable
					284	0.06		
					364	0.83		
					637	0.07		
^{123}I	^{121}Sb(α,2n)^{123}I	13 h	EC, γ	–	**159**	0.83	^{123}Te	1.2×10^{13} years
					27	0.72		
					31	0.15		
^{133}Xe	^{235}U(n,f)^{133}Xe	5 days	β⁻, γ	110.1	**81**	0.37	^{133}Cs	Stable
					31	0.40		
^{201}Tl	^{203}Tl(d,2n)^{201}Pb ^{201}Pb (9.33 h) → ^{201}Tl	72 h	EC, γ	–	X-ray[a] **70–80**	0.93	^{200}Hg	Stable
^{99}Mo	^{235}U(n,f)^{99}Mo ^{98}Mo(n,λ)^{99}Mo	67 h	β⁻, γ	390.1	140	0.82	^{99m}Tc	6 h
					740	0.14	^{99}Tc	2.1×10^5 years
					41			
^{89}Sr	^{88}Sr(d,p)^{89}Sr	51 days	β⁻	**583.1**	909	100	^{89}Y	Stable
^{57}Co	^{56}Fe(d,n)^{57}Co	270 days	EC, γ		**122**	0.86	^{57}Fe	Stable
					136	0.11		
^{81m}Kr	^{81}Rb → ^{81m}Kr	13 s	IT, γ		**190**	0.67	^{81}Kr	2.1×10^5 years
^{18}F	^{18}O(p,n)^{18}F	109 min	β⁺	242.1	**511**[b]		^{18}O	Stable
^{15}O	^{14}N(d,n)^{15}O	124 s	β⁺	735.1	**511**[b]		^{15}N	Stable
^{13}N	^{10}B(α,n)^{13}N	10 min	β⁺	491.1	**511**[b]		^{13}C	Stable
^{11}C	^{11}B(p,n)^{11}C	20 min	β⁺	385.1	**511**[b]		^{11}B	Stable
^{82}Rb	^{82}Sr → ^{82}Rb	76 s	β⁺	1409.1	**511**[b]		^{82}Kr	Stable

Source: Browne E, Firestone RB. *Table of Radioactive Isotopes*. New York: Wiley, 1986.

Bold print refers to medically important decay emissions for imaging, counting, or therapy.

[a]X-rays emitted following electron capture.

[b]Annihilation photons.

Essentials of Nuclear Medicine Physics and Instrumentation, Third Edition. Rachel A. Powsner, Matthew R. Palmer, and Edward R. Powsner.

© 2013 John Wiley & Sons, Ltd. Published 2013 by John Wiley & Sons, Ltd.

APPENDIX B

Major Dosimetry for Common Radiopharmaceuticals

Radiopharmaceutical	Effective dose (mSv/MBq) adult	Principal target organ dose (mGy/MBq (rad/mCi))
^{99m}Tc-DMSA (dimercaptosuccinic acid)	0.0088	Kidneys: 0.18 (0.666)
^{99m}Tc-HMPAO (ceretec)	0.0093	Kidneys: 0.034 (0.126)
^{99m}Tc-RBC	0.007	Heart: 0.023 (0.0851)
^{99m}Tc-MAG3 (mertiatide, mercaptoacetyl glycine3)	Normal renal function: 0.007 Reduced renal function: 0.0061	Bladder: 0.11 (0.407) Bladder: 0.083 (0.307)
^{99m}Tc nonabsorbable (such as DTPA or SC) for oral gastric emptying	Liquid: 0.019 Solids: 0.024	Upper lower intestine: 0.12 (0.444) Upper lower intestine: 0.12 (0.444)
^{99m}Tc pertechnetate	0.013	Upper lower intestine: 0.057 (0.211)
^{99m}Tc-DTPA (pentetate)	0.0049	Bladder: 0.062 (0.229)
^{99m}Tc-IDAs (iminodiacetic acid gallbladder imaging agents)	0.017	Gallbladder: 0.11 (0.407)
^{99m}Tc-MAA (macroaggregated albumin)	0.11	Lung: 0.066 (0.244)
^{99m}Tc-MDP and HDP	0.0057	Bone surface: 0.063 (0.233)
^{99m}Tc-Myoview (tetrofosmin)	Rest: 0.0076 Exercise: 0.007	Gallbladder: rest: 0.036 (0.133) Gallbladder: exercise: 0.027 (0.100)
^{99m}Tc-labeled large colloids (such as sulfur colloid)	0.0094	Spleen: 0.075 (0.278)
^{99m}Tc-Sestamibi	Rest: 0.009 Exercise: 0.0079	Gallbladder: 0.039 (0.144) Gallbladder:0.033 (0.122)
^{99m}Tc-WBC (HMPAO)	0.011	Spleen: 0.15 (0.555)
^{111}In-Octreotide	0.054	Spleen: 0.57 (2.11)
^{111}In-WBC	0.36	Spleen: 5.5 (20.4)[a]
^{111}InCl-DTPA[a] (intrathecal)	0.14	Spinal column: 0.95 (3.52)
^{123}I-MIBG (meta-iodobenzylguanidine)	0.013	Liver: 0.067 (0.248)
^{123}I Sodium iodide[a]	5% uptake: 0.038 15% uptake: 0.075 25% uptake: 0.11	Thyroid 5% uptake: 0.63(2.33) Thyroid 15% uptake: 1.9 (7.03) Thyroid 25% uptake: 3.2 (11.8)
^{131}I NP-59 (6-B- iodomethyl-19- norcholesterol)	1.8	Adrenals: 3.5 (13)
^{131}I Sodium iodide[a]	5% uptake: 2.3 15% uptake: 6.6 25% uptake: 11	Thyroid: 5% uptake: 72 (266) Thyroid: 15% uptake: 210 (777) Thyroid: 25% uptake 360 (1330)
^{133}Xe (xenon gas) rebreathing for 5 min[a]	0.0008	Lungs: 0.0011 (0.00407)
^{18}F-FDG	0.019	Bladder: 0.16 (0.592)
^{201}Tl (thallous chloride)	0.22	Kidneys: 0.48 (1.78) Ovaries 0.73 (2.70)

[a]Adapted from ICRP, 1988. *Radiation Dose to Patients from Radiopharmaceuticals*, ICRP Publication 53, ICRP Publication 53. Ann. ICRP 18(1–4)

Adapted from ICRP, 1998. *Radiation Dose to Patients from Radiopharmaceuticals (Addendum to ICRP 53)*, ICRP Publication 80. Ann. ICRP 28(3).

Essentials of Nuclear Medicine Physics and Instrumentation, Third Edition. Rachel A. Powsner, Matthew R. Palmer, and Edward R. Powsner.
© 2013 John Wiley & Sons, Ltd. Published 2013 by John Wiley & Sons, Ltd.

APPENDIX C

Sample Calculations of the S Value

Table C.1 lists the terms (variables) that are used to calculate the S value.

Example 1

The following is an example of the calculation of the S value when the target organ is the thyroid and the source organ is also the thyroid, after ingestion of ^{131}I for treatment of hyperthyroidism. To simplify the calculation, we have assumed that the thyroid concentrates 100% of the dose instantaneously, and we shall use only the photons and beta particles that contribute the most to the S value. In essence, as shown in Table C.2, an S value is calculated for each particle and photon, and these are summed into a total S value.

The total calculated S value of 1.93×10^{-2} is a fair approximation to the published value [1] of 2.2×10^{-2}. Our calculated value is based on a subset of the photons and particles and a gland size of 20 g.

Table C.1 Terms used in the calculation of the S value

Term	SI unit	Traditional unit	Description
E = energy of emissions	eV	MeV	Energy of particle(s) and/or photon(s)
n = number of emissions	1/Bq s		Abundance of photons or particles produced during each atom disintegration
K = constant for correction of units in equation	–	–	For the traditional units in this example, $K = 2.13$; for SI units, $K = 1$
Δ = equilibrium dose constant	kg Gy/Bq s	g rad/μCi h	Energy (E) times abundance (n) for each particle or photon times K
ϕ = absorbed fraction	–	–	Fraction of photon or particle energy absorbed by target
m = mass	kg	g	Estimated mass of target organ
Φ = specific absorbed fraction	1/kg	1/g	Absorbed fraction (ϕ) divided by mass of organ (m)
S (target source) = S value	Gy/Bq s	rad/μCi h	Mean absorbed dose to target organ for each unit of cumulated activity in source organ

Essentials of Nuclear Medicine Physics and Instrumentation, Third Edition. Rachel A. Powsner, Matthew R. Palmer, and Edward R. Powsner.
© 2013 John Wiley & Sons, Ltd. Published 2013 by John Wiley & Sons, Ltd.

Table C.2 Calculation of S value for thyroid as source and target

Emission	Mean number of emissions per disintegration (n)	Mean energy of emissions (MeV)	Equilibrium dose constant (Δ) (g rad/µCi h)	Absorbed dose fraction (φ) for thyroid as source and target organ	Specific absorbed dose (Φ) for a 20 g thyroid (g⁻¹)	S-factor (Δ × Φ) (rad/µCi h)
β^-_1	0.0080	0.2893	0.0048	1.0	0.05	2.4×10^{-4}
β^-_2	0.0664	0.0964	0.0136	1.0	0.05	6.8×10^{-4}
β^-_3	0.8980	0.1916	0.3666	1.0	0.05	1.83×10^{-2}
γ_1	0.0578	0.2843	0.0350	0.0310	1.1×10^{-4}	3.85×10^{-6}
γ_2	0.8201	0.3644	0.6366	0.0313	1.1×10^{-4}	7.00×10^{-5}
γ_3	0.0653	0.6367	0.0886	0.0313	1.1×10^{-4}	9.74×10^{-6}
γ_4	0.0173	0.7228	0.0267	0.0305	1.1×10^{-4}	2.90×10^{-6}
					Total S =	$\mathbf{1.93 \times 10^{-2}}$

Source: Data from Weber DA, Eckerman KF, Dillman LT, Ryman JC. *MIRD Radionuclide Data and Decay Schemes*. New York: Society of Nuclear Medicine, 1989; and Snyder WS, Ford MR, Warner GG, Fisher HL. MIRD supplement #3. Estimates of absorbed fractions for monoenergetic photon sources uniformly distributed in various organs of a heterogeneous phantom. Pamphlet 5. *J Nucl Med* 1969; 10:13 (Appendix A).

Table C.3 Calculation of S value for thyroid as source and kidney as target

Emission	Mean number of emissions per disintegration (n)	Mean energy of emissions (MeV)	Equilibrium dose constant Δ (g rad/µCi h)	Absorbed dose fraction for thyroid as source organ and kidneys as target organs (φ)	Specific absorbed dose (Φ) for 284 g kidneys	Individual S-factors (Δ × Φ) (rad/µCi h) for each emission
β^-_1	0.0080	0.2893	0.0048	0.0	0.0	0.0
β^-_2	0.0664	0.0964	0.0136	0.0	0.0	0.0
β^-_3	0.8980	0.1916	0.3666	0.0	0.0	0.0
γ_1	0.0578	0.2843	0.0350	4.23×10^{-5}	1.49×10^{-7}	5.22×10^{-9}
γ_2	0.8201	0.3644	0.6366	5.07×10^{-5}	1.78×10^{-7}	1.13×10^{-7}
γ_3	0.0653	0.6367	0.0886	7.44×10^{-5}	2.62×10^{-7}	2.32×10^{-8}
γ_4	0.0173	0.7228	0.0267	8.03×10^{-5}	2.82×10^{-7}	7.53×10^{-9}
					Total S value =	$\mathbf{1.48 \times 10^{-7}}$

The calculated total S value of 1.48×10^{-7} somewhat overestimates the published value of 1.4×10^{-7}.

Example 2

The dose to the kidneys from the thyroid in the same case as above is calculated in a similar manner in Table C.3, except that beta particle emissions do not contribute to the absorbed dose in the kidney. All particulate radiations (such as alpha and beta) are called **nonpenetrating** (see Chapter 3); they travel a very short distance, and all their energy is absorbed in the source organ. Photons (gamma and X-ray) are called **penetrating** radiation; they generally travel long distances and deposit energy outside the source organ. The value of ϕ for nonpenetrating radiation, ϕ_{np}, is equal to 1.0 if the target and source organ are the same (as in the example above), and $\phi_{np} = 0$ if the target organ is different from the source organ.

Reference

1. Snyder WS, Ford MR, Warner GG, Watson SB. *Absorbed Dose Per Unit Cumulated Activity for Selected Radionuclides and Organs*, MIRD Pamphlet No. 11 "S". New York: Society of Nuclear Medicine, 1975.

APPENDIX D

Guide to Nuclear Regulatory Commission Publications

Title 10, "Energy," Code of Federal Regulations (10CFR) [1]

Title 10 of the Code of Federal Regulations contains the regulations governing the use of nuclear materials by all individuals and organizations with a Nuclear Regulatory Commission (NRC) license. Three parts of this document are relevant to the practice of nuclear medicine: Part 19: Notices, Instructions, and Reports to Workers: Inspection and Investigations; Part 20: Standards for Protection against Radiation; and Part 35: Medical Use of Byproduct Material.

NUREG-1556, Vol. 9, Revision 2, Consolidated Guidance About Materials Licenses [2]

This document is a detailed guide for filling out an NRC license application for the medical use of radionuclides. The appendices I–W contain model procedures for several of the regulations outlined in 10CFR Parts 20 and 35.

Sections of these documents relating to routine practice are organized for reference in Table D.1.

Table D.1 Selected sections of 10CFR Parts 19, 20, and 35 and NUREG-1556, Vol. 9

Topic	10CFR Part.Section	NUREG-1556, Vol. 9, Revision 2 Model Procedures
Required posting of NRC Form 3 "Notice to Employees" and 10CFR Parts 19 and 20	19.11	
Required instructions to workers concerning risks associated with exposure to radiation	19.12	Appendix J
Requirement for reporting exposure data to individual workers	19.13	
Definitions of terms for Part 20	20.1003	
Development of radiation protection program to comply with regulations and ALARA	20.1101	Appendix N includes model spill cleanup procedures and other emergency procedures. Appendix T includes rules for wearing gloves, monitoring hands, labeling syringes, etc.
Occupational dose limits for adults	20.1201	

Essentials of Nuclear Medicine Physics and Instrumentation, Third Edition. Rachel A. Powsner, Matthew R. Palmer, and Edward R. Powsner.
© 2013 John Wiley & Sons, Ltd. Published 2013 by John Wiley & Sons, Ltd.

Table D.1 (*Continued*)

Topic	1OCFR Part.Section	NUREG-1556, Vol. 9, Revision 2 Model Procedures
Occupational dose limits for minors	20.1207	
Dose equivalent to embryo/fetus	20.1208	
Public dose limits	20.1301	
Minimum exposure threshold for monitoring individual workers	20.1502	
Requirement for room ventilation or other controls to reduce inhalation of airborne radiation	20.1701 or 20.1702	
Security and surveillance of radioactive materials	20.1801 and 20.1802	
Requirements for posting radiation signs	20.1901, 20.1902	
Requirements for receiving and opening packages	20.1906	Appendix P
Rules for waste disposal	20.2001	
Record keeping for individual monitoring results	20.2106	
Written directives with procedures for administration	35.40 and 35.41	Appendix S
Training requirements for radiation safety officers, medical physicists, authorized users, and nuclear pharmacists	35.50–35.59	
Use and calibration of the dose calibrator	35.60	
Calibration of survey instruments	35.61	Appendix K
Requirements for possession of sealed sources	35.67	Appendix Q includes model procedures for leak testing
Labeling of vials and syringes	35.69	
End-of-day surveys	35.70	Appendix R
Criteria for release of individuals following radioactive doses	35.75	Appendix U includes dose calculations for release of patients receiving therapeutic radionuclides
Use of unsealed radioactive materials for imaging studies for which no written directive is required	35.200	
Training requirements for imaging and localization studies	35.290	
Use of unsealed radioactive materials for which a written directive is required	35.300	
Training requirements for use of unsealed radioactive material for which a written directive is required	35.390	
Records of written directives and procedures for administration	35.2040 and 35.2041	
Dose calibrator calibration records	35.2060	
Radiation survey instrument calibration records	35.2061	
Records for unsealed source patient doses	35.2063	
Records for leak test and inventory of sealed sources	35.2067	
End-of-day survey records	35.2070	
Records for release of individuals containing radioactive materials	35.2075	

References

1. US Nuclear Regulatory Commission. Title 10, *Energy*, Code of Federal Regulations (10CFR), Office of the Federal Register, National Archives and Records Administration. Washington, DC: US Government Printing Office, Revised January 1, 2009.

2. US Nuclear Regulatory Commission. *Consolidated Guidance About Materials Licenses: Program-Specific Guidance About Medical Use Licenses*, Final Report, NUREG-1556, Vol. 9, Rev. 2. Washington, DC: Office of Federal and State Materials and Environmental Management Programs, US Nuclear Regulatory Commission, January 2008.

APPENDIX E

Recommended Reading by Topic

Basic Nuclear Medicine Physics and Instrumentation

Cherry SR, Sorenson JA, Phelps ME. *Physics of Nuclear Medicine*, 4th edn. Saunders, 2012.

Knoll GF. *Radiation Detection and Measurement*, 3rd edn. Hoboken, NJ: John Wiley and Sons, 2000.

PET and SPECT Technology

Wernick MN, Aarsvold JN. *Emission Tomography: The Fundamentals of PET and SPECT*. London: Elsevier, 2004.

CT Technology

Goldman LW. Principles of CT and CT technology. *J Nucl Med Technol* 2007; 35:115–128.

Goldman LW. Principles of CT: Multislice CT. *J Nucl Med Technol* 2008; 36:57–68.

DICOM and Information Technology

Pianykh OS. *Digital Imaging and Communications in Medicine (DICOM): A Practical Introduction and Survival Guide*. Springer, 2010.

NEMA Medical Imaging and Technology Alliance. Resource page: http://medical.nema.org/.

Nuclear Medicine Quality Control

Zanzonico P. Routine quality control of clinical nuclear medicine instrumentation: A brief review. *J Nucl Med* 2008; 49:1114–1131.

Radiobiology

Hall EJ, Giaccia AJ. *Radiobiology for the Radiologist*, 7th edn. Philadelphia: Wolters Kluwer/Lippincott, Williams, and Wilkins, 2012.

Mettler FA, Upton AC. *Medical Effects of Ionizing Radiation*, 3rd edn. Philadelphia: Saunders Elsevier, 2008.

ICRP. *The 2007 Recommendations of the International Commission on Radiological Protection*, ICRP Publication 103, Annals of the ICRP, 37(2–4). ICRP, 2007.

Radiation Dosimetry

Stabin MG. *Fundamentals of Nuclear Medicine Dosimetry*. New York: Springer, 2008.

Stabin MG. *Radiation Protection and Dosimetry*. New York: Springer, 2010.

Stabin MG. *RADAR—The Radiation Dose Assessment Resource*, http://www.doseinfo-radar.com/.

NRC Regulations

Siegel JA. *Guide for Diagnostic Nuclear Medicine and Radiopharmaceutical Therapy*. Reston, VA: Society of Nuclear Medicine, 2004.

Radiation Accidents

Oak Ridge Institute for Science and Education. *The Medical Aspects of Radiation Incidents*. Oak Ridge, TN: Radiation Emergency Assistance Center/Training Site (REAC/TS), http://www.orise.orau.gov/reacts, revised 4/19/2011.

Essentials of Nuclear Medicine Physics and Instrumentation, Third Edition. Rachel A. Powsner, Matthew R. Palmer, and Edward R. Powsner.
© 2013 John Wiley & Sons, Ltd. Published 2013 by John Wiley & Sons, Ltd.

Index

absorbed dose (D̄), 198–199
absorbed energy (H), 185
absorption, 23
accuracy, dose calibrator, 168
afterglow, 123
air calibration, 181
ALARA principle, 205
alpha decay, 9
alpha particles, 9, 25–28, 46, 212–213, 216–217
amplifiers, 61
Anger cameras, 73
angle of acceptance, 77
annihilation coincidence detection, 103
annihilation peak, 66
annihilation reaction, 9, 27, 104
antineutrinos, 9, 12
area monitors, 70
atomic number (Z), 7–8
attenuation, 22–24, 148
    contrast agents, 131
    correction, 114, 131–132, 148–149
    in HU, 125
    PET, 112–114
axial scanning, 123

background radiation, 205
backprojection, 134–136
    artifacts, 136, 140–141, 144–146
backscatter peak, 67
badge dosimeters, 53–57
bar phantoms, 172–173
bases in DNA, 186
beam hardening, 24
becquerel (Bq), 16, 18
beta decay, 9
beta particles, 9, 12, 25–29, 46, 213, 216–217

biological half-life (T_b), 197
blank scans, 179
blood counts, following radiation exposure, 218
body-contouring orbits, 94
bone scans, 86
breast-feeding and radionuclides, 209
breathing artifacts, PET-CT, 130–131
bremsstrahlung, 29, 119
buffer zones decontamination rooms, 214
Butterworth filters, 147

calibration, energy spectrum, 61, survey meters, 169,
    well counters and thyroid probes, 170
cameras, Anger, 73
    PET, 105, PET quality control, 177–181
    planar, quality control, 170–175
    SPECT, 91, 97, quality control, 175–177
cancer risk, 192, 193–194
cell cycle and radiosensitivity, 189
cells, and radiation, 185–192
center of rotation (COR), 175–177
central nervous system and cardiovascular syndrome,
    220
ceramic scintillators, CT, 123
chain reaction, nuclear reactor, 36
Chang algorithm, 148
characteristic lead X-ray peak, 67
charge, 1
chromosomes, 186
    radiation damage, 187–189, 219
circular orbits, 94
coincidence detection, 103–105, 109–110
coincidence peak, 66
collimators, 73–79, 103, 121
combination filters, backprojection, 147
Compton electrons, 21, 63

Essentials of Nuclear Medicine Physics and Instrumentation, Third Edition. Rachel A. Powsner, Matthew R. Palmer, and Edward R. Powsner.
© 2013 John Wiley & Sons, Ltd. Published 2013 by John Wiley & Sons, Ltd.

Compton peak (edge), 63–64
Compton scattering, 21, 67
computed tomography (CT), 122–126
    dosimetry, 201–202
    hybrid systems, 129–132, 149
    image displays, 153–158
    QC, 181–182
confidentiality, 161–162
constancy, dose calibrators, 168, survey meters, 169
contamination, 208, 214–216
    internal, 207–208, 221
continuous acquisition, 94
contrast agent artifacts, 131–132
contrast enhancement, 153–156
converging collimators, 78–79
coronal view, 152–153
Coulomb force, 1
count, 16
crystals, 60, 79, 107–108
    defect, 172
CT see computed tomography
CT numbers, 125, 154, 181–182
CTDI$_{vol}$, 201–202
cumulated activity (Ã), 198
curie (Ci), 16, 18
cutoff frequency, 147
cyclotrons, 35, 38

data handling, 161–166
data protection, 161–162
de-excitation, 6, 26
decay equation, 16
decay notation, 15–16
decay time of crystals, 67–68, 107
decontamination, 208, 214–216
    internal, 221
decorporation, 221
depth-of-interaction effect, 112
detectors
    gas-filled, 41–52
    luminescent, 54–57
    photographic, 53–54
    scintillation, 60–70
    semiconductors, 52–53
DICOM standard, 162–163, 165–166
digitization of images, 83–86
distance (exposure), 206–207, 217
diverging collimators, 79
DLP (dose length product), 201–202
DMWL (DICOM modality worklist), 165–166
DNA, 186–189, 191
doping of crystals, 60
dose calibrators, 48, quality control, 168–169
dose equivalent (H), 185
dose limits, 205–209

dose-related risk, 193
dosimeters, 49, 53–57, 70, 209, 217–218
dosimetry, 197–202, 225
dry desquamation, 221
dynamic imaging, 86–88
dynamic range, 153

edge-enhancing filters, 140–141
effective dose (E), 200, 202
effective half-life (T$_e$), 197
efficiency of detectors, 68–69, 170
elastic scattering, 213–214
electron binding energy, 4
electron capture, 12–14
electron volt (eV), 4
electrons, 4–6
    see also beta particles
elements, 1–3
elliptical orbits, 94
embryos, 192
emission scans, 179–181
employee safety, 205, 206–209, 217
energy spectrum (NaI crystals), 61–67
energy test, PET, 177
energy window, 61, 170
equilibrium, in generators, 32–35
erythema, 220, 221
excitation, 6, 25, 60
exposure, limiting, 205–209, 217–218

family members, exposure, 209
fan beam collimators, 79
fetal radiosensitivity, 192
film badges, 53–54
filtered backprojection, 134–136
    frequency domain, 141–148
    spatial domain, 136–141
fission, 9, 35–36
flood field uniformity, 170–172
flood uniformity correction, 175
[18]F-fluorodeoxyglucose (FDG), 198, SUV and, 115–116
Fourier transformation, 142
free radicals, 189, 191
frequency domain, 141–148
frequency spectrum, 141–142
frisking probes, 216
full width at half-maximum (FWHM), 173
full width at tenth-maximum (FWTM), 173

gadolinium orthosilicate (GSO) crystals, 107
gamma cameras see cameras
gamma rays, 14, 21–25, 46, 213
gantries, 79, 129–130
GAP collimators, 73
gas amplification, 43–44

gas-filled detectors, 41–52, quality control and, 168–169
gastrointestinal bleeding scan, 88
gastrointestinal radiation damage, 212, 220
gated images, 87
Geiger counters, 43, 44–46, 50–52, 216–217
general public, exposure, 205, 209
generators, 32–35
genetic disease, 193
geometric efficiency, 46, 69
geometry, dose calibrators, 168–169
gray (Gy), 185

half-life ($T_{1/2}$), 16
    types, 197
half-value layer (HVL), 24
halogenated pyrimidines, 191
Hann filters, 147
heart
    axes, 153
    imaging, 87, 92, 97–100
helical scanning, 123–126
hematopoietic syndrome, 220
high-energy collimators, 78
high-pass filters, 146, 147
high-resolution collimators, 77
HLA typing, 218
hospital information systems (HIS), 164
hospital workers, 205, 217
hospitals' role in nuclear incidents, 214–221
Hounsfield units (HU), 125, 154, quality control and,
    181–182
household contacts, exposure, 209
hygiene measures, 208, 209

indium-111 (^{111}In), 17, 35, 38
information technology systems, 161–166
ingestion, limiting, 208
inhalation, limiting, 208
inherited disease, 193
initial activity (A_0), 198
Integrating the Healthcare Environment, 164–165
internal conversion, 14
internal exposure, 207–208, 221
interphase G_1/G_2, 189
iodine escape peak, 64
iodine-131 (^{131}I), 17, 78, 198, 209, 217
ionization, 25–27
ionization chambers, 43, 46–49
ionization region, 43
isobars, 8
isomeric transition, 14
isotones, 8
isotopes, 8
iterative reconstruction, 149–152

k factors, 202
kinetic energy, 36

LD$_{50}$ of radiation, 192
light yield of crystals, 107–108
line of response (LOR), 103
line spread function, 172–173
linear attenuation coefficient (μ), 23
linear energy transfer (LET), 27, and DNA damage, 187,
    189–190, 212
linear no-threshold (LNT) hypothesis, 194
linearity
    CT number, 182
    dose calibrators, 168
    gamma cameras, 173
liver, imaging, 93–94
local area networks (LAN), 161–162
low-energy all-purpose (LEAP) collimators, 73, 77
low-pass filters, 146–148
luminescent detectors, 54–57
lung, radiation damage, 212
lutetium orthosilicate (LSO) crystals, 107–108
lymphocytes, 192, 218, 219

mass attenuation coefficient (μ/p), 23
mass defect, 7
matrices, 84–85
maximum intensity projection (MIP), 156
maximum likelihood expectation maximization (MLEM),
    150
medium-energy collimators, 78
MIRD system, 198–199
mitosis, 186, 189
modulation transfer function, 175
moist desquamation, 221
molecules, 1
monitoring of employees, 208–209
MPPS (modality performed procedure step), 166
multiplanar reformatting, 152–153
multislice CT scanners, 123
mutation rate, 193

nausea, 218
neon signs, 46
networks, 161–162, 163
neutrinos, 9
neutron capture, 36–38
neutrons, 6–7, 8, 35–36, 213–214
nine-point smoothing, 137–139
nitroimidazoles, 191–192
noise, 137–139, 144–148, 181
nonpenetrating radiation, 25
nonstochastic risks, 193
nuclear binding energy, 7

nuclear fission, 9, 35–36
nuclear incidents, 212–221
Nuclear Regulatory Commission (NRC), 205, 209, 228–229
nucleus (atomic), 4, 6–8
    unstable, 9–18
Nyquist frequency, 144

occupational exposure, 205, 206–209, 217
orbitals, 5–6
ordered subsets expectation maximization (OSEM), 150–152
organ toxicity, 192
oxygen as radiosensitizer, 191

PACS system, 163
pair production, 21, 66
pancake probes, 216
parallax error, 112
parallel-hole collimators, 73, 77–78
patient exposure, 209
patient motion artifacts, 97, 130
patient positioning, hybrid systems, 129
patients, management in nuclear incidents, 214–216, 218–221
peak applied voltage (kVp), 119
penetrating radiation, 25
periodic table, 3
persistence scopes, 83
personal protective equipment, 208, 217
PET see positron emission tomography
phantoms, 177, 181–182, bar, 172
photodiodes, 123
photoelectric effect, 21, 64, 67
photographic detectors, 53–54
photomultiplier tubes (PMT), 60–61, 79, 83, 108
    QC, 172, 179–181
photons see gamma rays; X-rays
photopeak, 63, 170
physical half-life (T_p), 197
pinhole collimators, 79
pitch, CT scans, 125
pixels, 84–86, 144
planar imaging, 86–88, QC and, 170–175
pocket dosimeters, 41, 49, 217
positioning algorithm, 79, 83
positron emission tomography (PET), 103–116
    PET-CT, 114, 129, 132, 149
    QC, 177–181, 182
positrons, 9–12, 27, 111
preamplifiers, 61
prefiltering, 147
pregnancy, 205, 209
projection views, 92–94

proportional counters, 43–44, 50
proportional region, 43
protons, 6–9, 12
pulse pileup, 68
pulse-height analyzers, 61, 83, 109

quality control (QC), 168–182, 217
quantum number, 5
quenching, 51

rad (radiation absorbed dose), 185
radiation, 9–14
    biological effects, 185–194
    interactions with matter, 21–29
radiation sickness, 218–221
radiation weighting factor (W_R), 185, 186
radioactive decay, 9–18
radiology information systems (RIS), 163–165
radionuclides, 107, 214, 224
    production, 32–38
radiopharmaceuticals, 105, 197–202, 225
radioprotectors, 192
radiosensitivity, 189, 192
radiosensitizers, 191–192
radium-226 (^{226}Ra), 17
ramp filters, 146, 147
random events, 105, 110
reactors, 35–38
rem (roentgen equivalent man), 185
renal scan, 87
residence time (τ), 198
resolution, 73, 77, 85–86
    CT, 182
    energy, 67
    evaluation, 172–175, 177, 182
    PET, 103–105, 110–112
risk, 192–194
roentgen (R), 48
Roentgen, Wilhelm, 119
rotate–rotate CT systems, 122–123
rotate–stationary CT systems, 122
rubidium-82 (^{82}Ru), 32, 33, 35, 111

S value, 198–199, 226–227
safety, 205–209, 217–218
sagittal view, 152–153
scintillation detectors, 60–70, QC and, 170
secular equilibrium, 33–35
self-dose, 199
semiconductor detectors, 52–53
sensitivity
    collimators, 73, 77
    gas-filled detectors, 46, 47, 51–52
    PET, 103, 111

septa
   collimators, 73, 77, 78
   PET, 110–111
shielding for radiation safety, 207, 217
sine waves, 141–144
single-photon emission computed tomography (SPECT),
      91–100
   QC, 175–177
   SPECT-CT, 129–132, QC and, 182
   3-D displays, 156–158
singles events, 103
sinograms, 97, 179
skin injury, 220, 221
slant-hole collimators, 78
smoothing technique, 137–139
sodium iodide (NaI) crystals, 60, 79, 107
source organ, 199
spatial domain, 136
spatial filtering, 137–141
specific ionization, 27
SPECT *see* single-photon emission computed tomography
spills, 208
spiral scanning, 123–126
standard uptake value (SUV), 115–116, QC and, 181
star artifacts, 136, 137
static imaging, 86
step-and-shoot acquisition, 94
stochastic risks, 192–193
subatomic particles, 4–18
surface rendering, 158
survey meters, 48, 50, 51, 70, QC and, 169, use in
      nuclear accidents, 214–217
synthetic (S) phase, 189

target organ, 68, 199
targets (production of radiation), 35, 36–38, 119
technetium-99m (^{99m}Tc), 17, 32, 33, 34, 198, 209
tenth-value layer (TVL), 24
thermoluminescent detectors, 55
3-D data displays, 156–158
3-D PET imaging, 111
thyroid probes, 69, QC and, 170
time (exposure), 206, 217

time of flight (PET), 105, QC and, 181
tissue effects of radiation, 192, 212–214
tissue weighting factor (W_T), 200–201
tomography, 91
total body dose, 200
transaxial slices, 134–136, 152
transient equilibrium, 32, 33
transmission attenuation correction, 114, 149
transmission scans, 177–179
transmutation, 38
treatment rooms, 214–215
triage score (T), 219
2-D PET imaging, 111

uniformity
   CT numbers, 182
   planar cameras, 170–172
   SPECT, 175

virtual private networks (VPN), 161–162
volume rendering, 158
vomiting and radiation exposure, 218
voxels, 153

well counters, 69–70, QC and, 170
white blood cells, 192, 218, 219
wide-area networks (WAN), 161
window, energy, 61
windowing (image contrast), 154–156
wipe tests, 68–69
worklist servers, 165–166
wounds, 215

X-linked diseases, 193
X-ray tubes, 119, QC and, 181
X-rays, 6, 67, 122
   bremsstrahlung, 29, 119
   characteristic, 25
   CT, 122–126
   production, 119–121
   tissue damage, 213

Z-pulse, 61, 83

Printed in the United States
By Bookmasters